Getting Through
to Difficult Kids and Parents

Getting Through to Difficult Kids and Parents

Uncommon Sense for Child Professionals

Ron Taffel

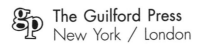

The Guilford Press
New York / London

To all my teachers

Library of Congress Cataloging-in-Publication Data

Taffel, Ron.
    Getting through to difficult kids and parents : uncommon sense for
child professionals / Ron Taffel.
        p. cm.
    Includes bibliographical references and index.
    ISBN 1-57230-475-8 (hc.)   ISBN 1-59385-093-X (pbk.)
    1. Social work with children.   2. Family social work.   3. Problem
children.   4. Problem families.   I. Title.

HV713.T27 2001
362.7—dc21   00-064043

About the Author

Ron Taffel, PhD, has supervised and written about working with children and families for over two decades, and is one of the country's most sought-after speakers for both professional and parent audiences. Dr. Taffel is the award-winning author of over 100 academic and popular articles, and has been a contributing editor to *McCall's* and *Parents* magazines for 10 years. His childrearing guides, translated into numerous languages, include the critically acclaimed *Parenting By Heart*, *Why Parents Disagree*, and *Nurturing Good Children Now*. He is the founder of Family and Couples Treatment Services at the Institute for Contemporary Psychotherapy in New York City, where he lives with his wife and two children.

Acknowledgments

I would like to thank Kitty Moore, my editor at The Guilford Press. While the following sentiment is pro forma for most acknowledgments, in this case it is true that without Kitty's encouragement, patience, and far-sightedness this book would absolutely never have been written. I don't remember working for such a long time on such a difficult project with such a smart, decent professional. My thanks as well to Bob Matloff, President, and Seymour Weingarten, Editor-in-Chief, at The Guilford Press, for embracing this project, and having the vision to see it through.

I would also like to thank my countless supervisors, among them Salvador Minuchin, Betty Carter, Dorothy Gartner, and Bernard Kalinkowitz, for helping me learn the different approaches I've integrated in these pages.

Very special thanks to Rich Simon, Editor-in-Chief of the *Family Therapy Networker*. Over the years he has encouraged me and provided me with a powerful forum. Rich's spirit and savvy are indirectly responsible for this work.

Finally, thanks to the Institute for Contemporary Psychotherapy, my professional home as a teacher, supervisor, and administrator these past two decades. Our modest not-for-profit training center has done a great deal to be proud of, having taught and helped thousands of people. As our 30th anniversary approaches, it's time to celebrate the Institute's accomplishments.

Preface

About 20 years ago I presented my first workshop to a PTA group. Because my training had been such an unusual amalgam—child development, adult analytic and family therapy—and because my professional experience had been so hands-on—director of treatment at an urban child psychiatric clinic, founder of family therapy at a not-for-profit training center, in addition to maintaining an extensive private practice—I struck a highly practical and, so it seems, inspirational note.

Word spread, and within a year I was doing approximately one seminar a week at many types of organizations. At the same time I had begun writing for a nonacademic professional magazine, the *Family Therapy Networker*, bringing my specific blend of clinical and practical approaches to a wide variety of professionals. It is difficult to believe now, but a significant number of my colleagues looked down on my atheoretical, pragmatic view of the work. For whatever reason, they did not seem to understand how much those on the front lines need help with basic techniques that increase the possibility of getting through to difficult kids and parents.

It wasn't hard for me to persevere, though. Child professionals of all types—counselors, teachers, school psychologists, caseworkers, pediatricians, nurses—were not shy about encouraging me. They deeply appreciated hearing about child development and parenting strategies. They were eager to learn concrete methods that would get kids to open up, help parents stay in charge, increase children's self-esteem, and encourage parents to create a united front.

My learning process continued. It entailed more than a thousand workshops with parents and child professionals covering the vast spectrum of children with special needs and ordinary daily challenges. Hearing from the adults in kids' lives prompted me to launch several studies with hundreds of "normal" kids and adolescents from a diverse socioeconomic population. Since I'd registered adult voices, I also wanted to learn about school children's thoughts and concerns: What matters most that parents do? How do kids feel about rules, rituals, and talking to adults? What small changes make a big difference? Finally, I participated in a wonderful study interviewing successful heterosexual and gay couples to determine what were the consistent themes of long-term relationship happiness.

This cumulative exposure to professional and family concerns again drove home the need for both pragmatism and vision. After all, for those 20-plus years I heard the same message. Line workers, parents, and kids kept reporting how drastically different our contemporary landscape is from the post-World War II, Victorian-based theories most of us were taught. I was reminded over and over that the demands on families are transforming daily, requiring professionals and parents to continuously reinvent themselves. My scope then gradually widened from individual children to families of all types and to the cultural forces at large.

*   *   *

A couple of years ago, I decided to write a book for professionals that would offer concrete techniques shaped by a coherent and up-to-date sociopolitical perspective. Since we all swim in the cultural seas, this book is not aimed at one kind of professional. Rather, it is based on an assumption born of many years' experience: the skills a teacher needs to get through to kids are not terribly different from the skills a caseworker or a pediatrician or a nurse or a counselor needs.

How should you approach this volume? As a child professional you are probably harried and have little time to waste. This book is written with such time constraints in mind. It is a no-nonsense presentation of just about everything you need to work with children and parents. It is written in a bare-bones way with many examples, so that *this week* you can apply a new understanding or concrete strategies to your work. And it is presented in an order that makes experiential sense to anyone who deals with kids and adolescents:

1. Making a good first contact with children and parents.
2. Spotting and diagnosing problem kids early on.
3. Getting through to difficult kids and adolescents.
4. Making a connection with difficult parents.
5. Handling one's own emotional reactions to intense situations.
6. Developing skills to strengthen kids' self-esteem and parents' effectiveness in setting limits.
7. Dealing with the extraordinarily challenging issues of modern teenagers.
8. Creating greater connectedness in fragmented families.
9. Building bridges between isolated parents, other families, and the school.

Though this is a comprehensive model, each chapter is presented in a step-by-step manner and is suitable for all professional contexts. Whatever your job description, have modest goals for yourself, just as you should with the kids and parents you meet.

*   *   *

Also, keep in mind that the suggestions I've made ought not to be tried if they don't feel consistent with who you are or if they are in conflict with your agency role or state guidelines. When in doubt, always check with your supervisor.

Remember, though, that these ideas are front-line tested and meant to be as realistic as possible. I understand what life is like for child professionals. I live it year after year and, like you, show up on the job every day. Society doesn't reward the work we do with the same kind of remuneration other (in my view) less essential services often command. But despite this, we keep trying, and in the process we need all the guidance we can get.

If this book makes you any more effective, helps you feel more connected to the kids and parents you deal with, or encourages you to feel a little more alive doing the work, it will have been worthwhile.

Contents

chapter one

Getting Started

How to Quickly Gather the Information That Counts

A child is the class clown, and his worried father comes to you for guidance.

A girl is extremely bossy with her playmates, and her mother is upset that fewer parents are calling to arrange get-togethers.

A boy is being scapegoated mercilessly by classmates. He is tormented for the way he looks and because he is smart. His mother and father are beside themselves.

This is where we begin. When parents approach us regarding children they want answers to help them understand what is going on and then concrete suggestions about what needs to be done. Nothing more, nothing less. Yet, unless we have time to visit a classroom or the home of a family, accurate information is hard to come by. This lack of data—being a *witness* to a child's actual behavior—creates a palpable division between parents and professionals. Without seeing kids in their milieu, it's almost impossible to sufficiently empathize with a mother or father.

Faced many times with the dilemma of being approached by

anxious parents who offer little information to guide me, I have developed a repertoire of techniques to uncover what is wrong with a child or family so that I can make effective suggestions. In this chapter I will outline the three information-gathering techniques that I have found to be adaptable in all professional roles—teachers, guidance counselors, clergy, and so on.

Enactments

Years ago, Salvador Minuchin, along with other therapists, developed a school of treatment called structural family therapy. When I learned this method, I never realized how simple it would be to use in all settings, nor how valuable it would be in helping diagnose children's difficulties and advising parents. During the last few decades, structural family therapy has become an integral part of the mental health field and the helping professions, especially when clinicians are working with highly disturbed populations. Yet, it is surprising to me that few professionals know how to implement its most powerful data-gathering technique—"the enactment."

The basic concept behind the enactment is that family members, if prodded to discuss a conflictual issue, invariably act out the most important dynamics that need to be focused on. While we may not have been formally taught this principle, we're familiar with it because enactments happen in our lives all the time. Borrowed originally from interpersonal psychoanalytic theory, "enactment" is really another way of saying that family members' patterns of responding to each other are so ingrained and reflexive they spontaneously appear, no matter how determined we are not to repeat them.

For example, Tom, an extremely successful chief executive officer of a multinational corporation, tells me, "It doesn't matter that I'm the head of a huge company. But when I visit my mother I'm still her youngest child and the baby of our family. Within a couple of minutes, no matter what I've decided beforehand, I feel stupid and start saying the kind of things that would get me immediately fired from my job."

We are all intuitively familiar with Tom's experience. Each time we visit the families we grew up in, it is almost impossible to avoid the same "dance" with mothers and fathers, sisters and brothers that we did when we were children or young adults. The enactment draws on this time-tested fact of family life: interactions, especially troublesome ones, are destined to repeat themselves. As an information-gathering technique, the enactment can thus be reliably used in almost any professional situation—say, a parent–teacher conference, when a guidance counselor must call in parents, or when a pastoral counselor sees a couple.

Setting Up an Enactment

1. Pick a topic. A child is having trouble doing homework. Or another won't pay attention to his parents. To begin an enactment, simply get a conversation going between parents and kids about the presenting problem. For example, ask mother and child to discuss homework or the latest disagreement. Say to the parents and child: "I'd like you to talk together about the way you do homework," "I'd like you, Mom, to talk with Johnny about the trouble you have getting him to pick up for himself around the house."

2. Prepare family members for a moment or two of self-consciousness. Even if they've known you for years, most people are self-conscious when they're asked to discuss personal matters in front of a non-family member. This awkwardness needs to be addressed. Say, "I know this will seem strange at first. But I guarantee in a few minutes, it will feel much more natural." Normalize by referring to the many other families with whom you've had experience with enactments (remember, in your personal life these interactions go on all the time—when you're on a double date, or with your kids at a big family dinner). Or, if you can't think of other examples, be honest and say, "I'd like to try a technique I've learned."

3. Make yourself as invisible as possible during the interaction. There are several ways to do this. Don't make eye contact with family members, since this leads to greater self-consciousness.

How? Lean back, literally face another direction or look down at your notes. From the beginning, the boundary expressed through your body language communicates that whatever goes on is the *family's* doing, not an artificial exchange created by being in your presence.

Making oneself "invisible" almost always works to relieve initial reluctance. After a few moments of feeling self-conscious, family members are off and running, engaged in the same interactive patterns that have taken place hundreds of times before their meeting with you.

What to Look for

Observe the most concrete behaviors, the basic steps in the family's dance. Do not interpret, and do not look for hidden motivation. Ask yourself questions that begin with words such as "what," "who," and "where." Do not get yourself stuck on asking "why" or "when." The following are some examples of what to look for:

• *Tone of voice*—respectful, contemptuous, and so forth. A nice-guy dad complains that his boy, James, is inexplicably a wise guy in school. Mom is also concerned about her son's negative attitude with other adults, with whom he constantly finds fault. During the enactment, this very nice man surprisingly speaks to his son in a derisive tone, especially when the boy disagrees with him. "I've never heard anything so ridiculous," he says. Dad's attitude infuriates his son and, in turn, the boy shouts, "Yeah? . . . You don't know anything either!" further aggravating the father.

• *Loudness*—who drowns out whom? In the Marion family, everyone had to yell to be heard. Katie, a fifth grader who had trouble standing up for herself in school, was unable to speak during the enactment. As everyone screamed at each other over every possible issue, Katie could not get a word in edgewise. In just a few minutes, it was clear where she had learned to be so reserved.

• *Reactivity*—the quickness and intensity of family members' responses to each other. Parents had complained about disagreements over the kids. They then demonstrated their endless fighting when the counselor got them to discuss a time for the next appointment. They were so inflamed that the counselor told me, "It was as if I didn't exist in the room."

- *Interrupting*—who does it to whom? I asked Danny and his mother to discuss bedtime. During the 5-minute conversation that ensued, Mom interrupted her son, by my count, 15 times. Danny had developmental language problems. The extra challenge this presented, when combined with Mom's impatience, painfully became clear during the enactment.

- *Listening*—who listens; who does not? Dad was a wonderful listener while the family discussed differences of opinion. Mom, on the other hand, lectured to their oppositional and sullen daughter. The more Dad listened, the more Mom said he was being too softhearted and launched into another lecture. During this interaction, Mom, who was just as concerned about her daughter's welfare, became "the bad guy" compared to ever-patient Dad.

- *Relatedness*—who's talking to whom; who's left out? A tough-guy father interrupted loudly, repeatedly barging into the conversation I got going about curfew for his adolescent son. Despite his ineffectiveness, Dad prided himself on being the family's teacher of life lessons. As the enactment went on, this tough guy was slowly pushed to the periphery. No one talked about anything without going through Mom; certainly no one listened to Dad as he barked and sputtered from the sidelines.

- *Leadership*—who speaks first? In some families, the person who speaks first during the enactment is a paper tiger. In others, this person sets the tone of the entire discussion. The latter was the case in the Johnson family. Whatever mood Dad was in seemed to set the stage for any discussion that followed. Enactments were merely a reflection of dad's predominant mood.

- *Closure*—who gets the last word; can a conclusion be reached? With Annie, a 14-year-old who was in trouble because of acting out in school, the enactment between her and her mom was very telling: Annie always had to get the last word in. Unfortunately, so did her mother. Keeping the enactments down to several minutes was next to impossible since, just like at home, they could never end their arguments. Each just got madder at the other and more determined to have the last word.

How to Keep Notes

As you are observing the interactions take notes, keeping them simple by using the headings in the accompanying box to guide you. Note taking also help create an invisible boundary allowing parents and kids to feel less conscious. Here is an example of simple but accurate note taking:

1. Child ignores parent.
2. Parent raises voice.
3. Child starts fidgeting and looking away.
4. Parent begins to scream.

When to Stop the Enactment

There is no exact time limit to the length of an enactment. However, in my experience, it usually lasts no more than 10 or 15 min-

---

What to Look For

Tone of voice

Loudness

Reactivity

Interrupting

Listening

Relatedness

Leadership

Closure

utes. Almost everything you need to know emerges within the first few moments of a family discussion. Because of this, there is no reason to let an enactment go on for very long. In the Muller family, for example, it immediately became clear that each time Mom asked Susie to do her homework, she would confront her daughter with a barrage of questions that only caused Susie to become sullen and uncooperative. The dance continued—the more Susie was sullen, the more her mom talked and lectured. As is often the case, this troubled interaction became apparent within a couple of minutes.

The only reasons to immediately stop an enactment are the following:

1. A family member is getting out of control, and you're concerned about physical danger. In the White family, tempers got so inflamed during the enactment that Dad actually got up from the chair and hovered menacingly over his 14-year-old daughter, screaming obscenities at her while tightening his fists. In a situation such as this, I always do whatever is necessary to stop the escalating exchange—a verbal directive, getting up myself, standing between family members. Actual physical attacks are, in my experience, extremely rare. I've only seen one—purposely shown on a teaching tape made for therapists, counselors, and school personnel—that got out of hand; this, during 20 years of doing and teaching family enactments.

2. A parent is so ineffective, you're concerned he or she will walk out from your meeting feeling terribly embarrassed. I was sitting with a smart-talking 11-year-old preteen boy. His arguments during the interactions were so foulmouthed that just a minute or two were enough to see the kind of trouble parent and child got into. When I asked his mom, Nancy, to begin talking about rules regarding his allowance and spending money, within 2 or 3 minutes, this boy was calling his mother "an asshole." To extend the enactment any longer would have been to further publicly shame his parent.

3. A child is being humiliated by an out-of-control adult. A girl with attentional and learning difficulties was in my office with her overachieving, intellectualized parents. The more questions they asked her, the more "dumb" this girl got. As her parents became increasingly impatient, words such as "lazy" and "stupid" were directed at her. It was enough. The enactment needed to be over. I had learned all I needed to know.

In short, there is no reason for extending an enactment if the result is physical danger or psychological humiliation to anyone.

Feedback: How Do You Give It?

The ability to find something positive is one of family therapy's greatest contributions to a mental health field steeped in pathologizing. To most teachers, guidance counselors, therapists and so on, it does not come easily—it is a skill borne of practice. The rules of positive feedback are as follows:

   1. Be positive. After family members have interacted in very personal ways, you must give them feedback that is both concretely useful and emotionally positive in nature. To illustrate, the Johnsons had just screamed at each other for 10 minutes over their difficulty organizing the nightly bedtime routine with the kids. Yet, despite the nasty exchange, I could also see how concerned they were about each other. With this in mind, I said, "Mom and Dad, you obviously care that your children get enough rest. Though this arguing may not be an effective way to resolve your differences, it is clear to me how seriously you take your job."

   2. Be brief. Long explanations are lost, overly intellectualized, or can't be implemented. Following is an example of feedback that proved to be useless to the parents I was advising. "When you speak in that tone to your child, it may be better than how your parents spoke to you, but it is still experienced by your son as more critical than you really want. Children at this age often, like your son, hear constructive criticism in a different way than we mean them. They just hear the critical tone, not the concern that exists behind it."

It may seem surprising that I would consider such a relatively brief statement as too complicated. However, the longer I work with families, the more respectful I am of how nervous parents are about whatever feedback is given to them. A good rule of thumb is to keep your comments down to one concept, one sentence, or one small suggestion.

This guideline would turn the above statement into: "Your comments show you care, but is you tone getting through?"

3. Get to "needs" beneath the more obvious anger and frustration. Most people come to professionals, especially front-line workers, teachers, guidance counselors, and agency therapists, with absolutely no motivation to change themselves. They are angry and in a mood to blame. Finger-pointing combined with expressions of disappointment and justifications for anger are the ways many present themselves. It is easy for you as a counselor to be intimidated or outraged if you don't hear the vulnerabilities that exist just beneath the angry surface. Clearly, the best professionals I know who work with children and families are able to focus on the underlying needs. For example, when Mary came in to meet her daughter's teacher, she could barely contain her anger at Katherine's lack of cooperativeness about her homework and her poor study habits. Listening carefully, this wise teacher was able to hear Mom's disappointment not only in her daughter but also in herself as a parent. The teacher's response addressed both Mom's frustration and the hidden hurt: "You need to be more assertive with your daughter because you'll feel better about yourself as a parent."

Another such example occurred when Ernest and Helene complained to their pediatrician about their inability to divide child care arrangements in a way that made both parents happy. Ernest was particularly enraged because, as he put it, "She is overinvolved with the child." After listening to both sides, this savvy pediatrician said to Ernest, "If you ask your wife more gently, she'll be more likely to give you the affection I think you really want."

4. Be balanced. In order to get family members ready for change, it is important to offer balanced feedback. This is extremely difficult. The outrage we often feel at what we perceive to be "unfair" behavior makes it likely that we attribute more blame to one or the other family member. Such judgments belie our hidden attitudes: women are hysterical; men can't communicate; kids are impossible; this couple shouldn't be together; and so on.

By balance I mean addressing different family members with an equal level of respect. Try not to sound authoritarian, especially like the self-important professional who knows it all. This is easier said than done. After all, a lot of mental health practices developed from an era informed by psychoanalysis, at a time when therapists were expected to decisively "nail" people with precise interpretations. Many professionals do not realize they come from this tradition, and they have a hard time keeping away from flashy but ultimately disrespectful communication. Provocative pronouncements such as "Your child has you wrapped around her finger" may be true, but the humiliation and shame such statements create often rupture a parent's relationship with you.

I found this out years ago. Once, sitting with a family, I was struck that during the enactment, each person seemed to protect the feelings of another family member. Instead of commenting on how sensitive they were toward each other, I came up with the pithy observation that their exchange reminded me of the way communication might sound in a well-mannered "protection racket." This was right on the money, but it was delivered in a curt, sarcastic tone that severed my connection with the family. Such statements make for dramatic showmanship and temporary satisfaction about being tough and confrontational, but they often mark the last time we will see a family.

Feedback that is more balanced makes a huge difference. Compare the statement "Your child has you wrapped around his finger" with "Your child is incredibly tenacious. It's no wonder that she has you wrapped around her finger." This direct but balanced feedback is exactly what helps family members feel understood. It subtly prepares them for the idea that the process of change is about *everyone* working on *something*. In this case, after commenting on the child's tenacity, it is easy to move toward suggestions that will be experienced empathically: "Since your daughter is so tenacious, we need to figure out ways together that can help you to be more in charge.

Because of her strong will, you might have to work harder than most parents."

Keep in mind the following rules about feedback:

- The problem is almost never one person's fault.
- You are not blaming anyone as being single-handedly responsible for any difficult interaction.
- You are doing your best to see the situation from everyone's point of view.
- Each person is part of a system that is interdependent and therefore everyone has to change a little.

Putting It Together

The enactment provides a practical, nonintrusive way to get to know parents and kids in a very short time, often yielding just the right kind of feedback to get parents started on the change process. Following is an example in which I've included the presenting problem, setting up the enactment, and giving positive, balanced feedback.

A 12-year-old girl, Amelia, was having difficulty keeping up in school as well as paying attention to her parents at home. Amelia's marks had declined so sharply that she was on the brink of being kicked out of junior high. She was referred to me by her teacher, a woman I'd met at a parenting workshop. I began an enactment with the family around a very "hot" family disagreement—the issue of curfew. Within just a few minutes, it was clear that her father, Bernie, who was the "disciplinarian," was getting nowhere with Amelia. Each time I asked Bernie to create a curfew, he would begin abstractly discussing the importance of following rules, respecting authority, listening to your elders, and the like. His daughter Amelia, if she wasn't offering lame or provocative excuses, quickly got that glazed, far-off look—a sure indication of a parent being tuned out. Dad did not seem to notice or care. Even with my gentle prodding that he try to specifically name a curfew, Bernie could not stop speaking in an abstract way: "How will you learn the

Feedback That Gets Through

UNBALANCED	BALANCED
"You don't understand your child."	"Your child is challenging and complex. It's not surprising how difficult she is to understand."
"You're yelling too much."	"Your child's stubborn, but yelling doesn't seem to be getting through either."
"You criticize a lot of the time."	"I know you're frustrated and that easily turns into criticism; it's difficult to know what to do with him in the moment."
"You need to listen better to your child."	"It's always hard when there are two spirited kids like these. You'll have to learn to listen to one at a time."
"As his parents, you've got to be more of a united team."	"Your family's so busy, it's just about impossible for the two of you to discuss and think through decisions . . ."

meaning of rules?" "What will become of you?" "Curfews may not seem important, but it's like any other job . . . "

This enactment revealed the self-defeating dance that Bernie and Amelia had fallen into. For reasons I would find out later, Bernie had tremendous difficulty getting specific about what he expected. Helping him to be clearer about his expectations was a direct result of my closely watching the interaction between father and daughter.

My feedback, in which I tried to be very balanced, particularly about dad's difficulty making himself heard, was the following:

"You've got a tough kid here who does need to learn a few life lessons. But I think you need to start a little smaller. Next time, see if you can get a specific time across in just one or two sentences." Our work then focused on helping Dad get more to the point with his daughter and not be sidetracked by her considerable skill at obfuscating. This was clearly aided by witnessing firsthand the interaction between them.

Stories from Home

Often we can't or shouldn't get a child immediately involved in our meetings with the parents, and certainly not engaged in an enactment. For the various reasons this occurs, I often ask parents to write brief "stories from home" focused on conflictual interactions around the house. When I first began doing this I encountered a lot of resistance, not from families but from professionals in the mental health field who did not like the idea that family members would be excluded. Teachers trained in modern philosophy of education believed that children should be present for all conferences. Guidance counselors, therapists, and family counselors were also hesitant to get "one-sided" information from the parents. Surprisingly, since many professionals have been taught that counselors must work with the whole family, they have been often surprised that there are good reasons why it may be better to meet with only the available parent(s).

The reason you may think it necessary that family work requires the presence of everyone is simple—that's the way family therapy used to be. In the late 1960s and early 1970s, therapists, just forging a new treatment of family "systems," were absolutely militant about the need for calling in every family member. Since families are systems, it was believed, if one part is left out the whole interaction is fundamentally altered. Theoretically, while there is some truth to this, in the real world it is often extremely difficult or even inadvisable to demand that every sibling or all family members who live in the house attend a meeting with you. In fact, over time, most counselors painfully learned that if they stuck to the "it's everyone or no one" rule of thumb, they often ended up working with no one.

There are several reasons to leave out some family members:

- Children refuse to come in with their parents to see you.
- A child is less than 5 years old; in these cases it is often easier to work primarily through the parents
- There are siblings involved who don't want to be dragged in or shouldn't be.
- The children's schedules are so crowded, time simply can't be found.
- You would like to delay a child's involvement because his parents believe that seeing a professional might hurt his self-esteem.

When you need to keep kids out of the diagnostic process, you're still faced with the problem of quickly gathering useful information. One of the most effective ways to uncover underlying issues without involving children is the technique of "writing stories."

The reason stories from home are so effective is, again, the power of "the dance" between family members. Regardless of a parent's psychological sophistication, it is astonishing how unaware most of us are about the repetitive and predictable steps that make up the family dance. This is why getting parents to write brief vignettes about difficult interactions around the house just about always reveals the information you'll need to know to give advice. The technique is particularly effective at getting concrete information about conflictual issues in a family's day-to-day life.

For example, Dierdre was having a lot of difficulty getting along with playmates; she always needed to be the boss; she wouldn't listen to her teacher and answered authorities back disrespectfully. For a variety of reasons, mostly having to do with Dierdre's brittle self-esteem, her teacher, Ms Smith, did not want to set up a school conference including Dierdre. To find out why Dierdre was having difficulty, I asked Ms Smith to enlist Mom's help by having her write about several scenarios around the house, focusing on areas of conflict such as Dierdre picking up after herself or getting ready for bed in the evening.

Guidelines for Writing Stories

Generally, it is important to keep these guidelines in mind when assigning this task:

1. Ask whether a parent anticipates trouble keeping a log. For example, someone might say, "I don't write well." Another might angrily object, "I already have too much work." Your response to these concerns is to reassure parents that the length or quality of the writing doesn't matter. Say: "I'm not interested in your presentation. Write it any way you want. I just need real-life material to help you figure out what to do."

2. Lighten the work load for pressured parents. Say: "Jot down a few notes after an incident, and make it brief. Just write, 'She said—I said—she said—I said,' and that's it!" Ask for a half dozen of these interactions, and once again remind parents that you're not doing this to make more work for them but to get first-hand material to help you make suggestions.

3. Ask the parent to read his or her stories out loud. The reason I ask parents to read vignettes firsthand is because only *they* know the proper inflection. In telling the story, their own feelings about the interaction become very apparent. They then take greater ownership of the incident. When parents hand me a copy of the stories that they've written from the week before, I always tell them the truth: "It would be more realistic if *you* read the story yourself."

In Dierdre's case, her mom, Elaine, came back a week later with a number of interactions in hand. Each one of them graphically described how ineffective Elaine was with bossy Dierdre in daily interactions around the house—homework, bedtime, picking up after herself. Here's an example:

MOM: I want you to pick up after yourself.

DIERDRE: (*Ignores mom and says nothing.*)

MOM: I'd like you to do it *now*.

DIERDRE: Not now, later. (*without looking up*).

MOM: If you don't pick up your clothes right now, I will take TV away from you for the entire year.

DIERDRE: So, go ahead . . . I don't care!

These unenforceable threats, which were repeated many times, over many different issues, made Elaine terribly ineffective as a parent. She felt abused by Dierdre and, on top of it, helpless because obviously her punishments were useless. As the pattern in these stories emerged, it quickly became clear to both Elaine and me that she needed to create smaller but enforceable consequences. This subsequent change in her ability to follow through profoundly affected life around the house.

4. One final matter to keep in mind. Many parents return saying "You know what? That thing we were talking about last week? It never happened. I had nothing to write about." This is not unusual and is actually a positive diagnostic sign. It means that, in some cases, a bit of self-reflection may in and of itself lessen conflictual interactions around the house. Don't be concerned though; the parents will need that ability to reflect once the dance inevitably reappears.

Tasks

A final way to gather information is to assign tasks for a parent to try at home. In figuring out what's wrong, task assignment is an extremely effective tool. The reason we assign "homework" is not to create change *but to actually see where the task fails*. Usually, how a parent has difficulty carrying out a homework assignment tells us exactly what underlying difficulties need to be addressed.

For example, Olivia, mother of two rambunctious teenage

boys, found it very difficult setting limits for both of her sons. This was a particular problem with 11-year-old Ethan. Since Olivia couldn't seem to find the time to write down stories and the boys refused to come in to see the counselor, I suggested that the counselor assign Olivia a homework assignment: "Whenever you and Ethan get into a heated argument and he steps out of line, try to leave—go to another room instead of continuing to fight with him."

The next week, Mom came back and said she had a difficult time *not* continuing the argument and, in fact, couldn't help herself from going after Ethan. Her reasons, it turned out, were specifically to try to get him to apologize for whatever his rudeness or infraction was. The counselor asked Olivia, "Why are you so intent on getting an apology from him?" At that point, Mom broke down and revealed to the counselor a secret: She had been chronically abused by her father and uncle. "For my whole life," sobbed Olivia, "all I ever wanted is for them to apologize to me for what they did."

Did the task fail? Only if your expectation had been to promote change. Much more importantly, it revealed the underlying problem. Olivia allowed herself to be drawn into these abusive interactions with her sons precisely because her *own* history of abuse drove her to seek the apology she'd never gotten. Once this became clear, the counselor could work much more easily toward helping Olivia disengage from useless power struggles with her boys.

Another example: Years ago, a couple, Florence and Buddy, came to see me about their constant disagreements over the kids and the resulting distance they felt toward each other. I assigned them the task of going out on a Saturday night date. Weeks later, having been unable to "find the time or make arrangements," Florence admitted something important—she was afraid of going out on a Saturday night knowing her infirm and totally dependent mother might suddenly need her. This was a worry she had never been able to openly discuss. Until the task "failed," Florence could not begin to make any changes regarding the real problem—her relationship with her mother—and certainly could not find time to make a date with her husband. That week we discussed Florence getting a telephone answering machine. The meeting centered on her feelings about such a device, the type of message to leave ("clear but not mean"), and how to tell her mom about this new addition to the house. Not exactly high-tech counseling, but extremely effective—and all garnered from the "failed" task.

Guidelines for Diagnostic Tasks

1. Pick an area the family wants to change. The most powerful way to find out what prevents change in a family is, to paraphrase George Bernard Shaw's observation, "Give them exactly what they want." So, if a presenting problem is that a couple doesn't have any downtime away from the kids, ask them to see if they can figure out a couple of hours to spend together during the next week. If a parent comes in saying that they have a hard time controlling their criticism over a child's eating habits, ask them to try to lay off for a week or two. In other words, to conceive of a homework assignment, use the person's motivation around a painful conflictual area.

2. Prepare them for failure. Obviously, if the family could manage to create such change on their own they wouldn't be coming to you in the first place. In order to maintain a relationship, it is essential to prepare them in an empathic way to realize that it will be very difficult to be successful. Normalize this by saying, "It's a one in a million shot that this is going to work. It's hard for anyone to change something that's been going on for such a long time." And tell family members not only to expect failure but to pay attention to what it is that gets in the way. For example, the couple without enough downtime was unable to come up with an hour or two to spend relaxing together. However, they returned to our next meeting with important information: they found no free moments to share because their schedules were at cross-purposes, making it highly unlikely that they would be at the same place, in the same mood, at the same time.

3. Reassure the client that your role is to help change. After such failure, it is easy for embarrassment and/or discouragement to set in. It is therefore extremely important to be direct and not lose hope yourself. Remember, the important point is that finding out *why* the family could not succeed at their task is a success. Being able to say, "I'm glad that this happened. Now I really know what you're up against," may be the most reassuring words a family can hear.

For example, Claudia, the mother of two boys 7 and 4 years old, came in overwhelmed because of the fights she was having with her younger son, Adam, over everything. "All I want to do," said Claudia, "is fight with him a lot less." As a diagnostic task, then, I assigned Claudia the job of trying to stay out of power struggles with Adam. I prepared her for the likelihood that this would be impossible and asked her to pay attention to what went wrong. Two weeks later Claudia returned, describing the task's failure in detail. But she was not at all discouraged. In the process of paying attention to their interactions, Claudia became significantly more aware of how tenacious both she and Adam were. Said Claudia, "For the first time I realized that not only is Adam relentless about getting what he wants but so am I." With this experiential truth now vividly noted, Claudia and I were able to start focusing on how she could begin to pick and choose her battles more wisely.

$$* \qquad * \qquad *$$

Using these three techniques to get information will help enormously. In almost every situation, they will quickly enable you to gather crucial material about what actually goes on between family members. In turn, you'll have the necessary information to offer concrete guidelines and suggestions to parents and kids.

Down and Dirty Diagnosis

chapter two

Spotting Developmental and Psychiatric Problems Early On

A girl won't eat in the lunchroom. Is she oppositional or does she have an eating disorder?

A boy talks very loud and stands too close to other kids. Does he have problems with his hearing, or is he simply bossy with peers?

A kindergartner often sits under the table in her classroom. Is she fearful or trying to get attention from the teacher?

A first-grade girl has tantrums when she doesn't get her way. Is she a spoiled brat or a child with more serious developmental difficulties?

Over the last 10 years, there has been an explosion in knowledge about child development and childhood psychiatric problems. Yet most child professionals, especially those on the front lines of daily child care—teachers, pediatricians, social workers, school counselors, therapists, preschool teachers, and so on—don't know how to spot psychiatric problems or delays in healthy child development. Nor have most of us been trained when and where to refer these children. Too often we ignore or, worse, misinterpret a child's behavior. We pejoratively label him as bad, oppositional, or perhaps spoiled. We attribute complex family or individual dynamics, implicating the parents in malevolent or negligent behavior.

While of course there may be truth to our conclusions, many kids have some developmental delay, or what I call psychophysiological disorder, which needs to be addressed. Unfortunately, because most of us are not trained in picking up early warning signals, these kids go on in their development without being sent to the appropriate specialist for help. Over time, children tend to *become* their inaccurate labels: They *do* act out! They *are* oppositional! They *do* seek attention! By adolescence, which is when I most often meet such kids, they are in deep trouble. Major behavioral problems have developed, which turn out to have been avoidable if only the signals had been caught earlier.

It is therefore incumbent for child professionals to pick up on certain signs and be aware of the need to consider referral to a specialist. This chapter is not an officially sanctioned diagnostic handbook. Rather, it is a working guide of everyday signals to notice; ordinary, parent-friendly questions to ask; and appropriate professionals to consult. I have divided each section into four parts that take into account the kinds of signs professionals in different settings will be able to pick up on:

1. The everyday signals of underlying issues
2. The way behaviors are often misinterpreted
3. Simple questions to ask parents
4. Where to refer a child

Pervasive Developmental Disorder

One of the more serious problems in child development, in modern clinical usage pervasive developmental disorder (PDD) is considered to be on a continuum that ranges from autism at the most extreme end to delayed development—which often improves over time and with the proper interventions—at the other. What many helping professionals might miss is that the signs of PDD manifest themselves very subtly and that early intervention with children even as young as 2 and 2½ years of age can be extremely helpful, if not life altering.

PDD manifests in three distinct areas of development. If a child has disturbances in all three areas, it is a good indicator of a pervasive disorder. The three areas are *language development*; *relatedness* (i.e., the ability to connect with parents and peers), and *sensory defensiveness*, which, loosely translated, means discomfort with different types of external stimuli.

Language Development

Disturbances in Receptive Language

Receptive language processing is the ability to take in and receive language and to organize and make meaning of what is heard. Disturbances in receptive language processing are the earliest signals of delays in language development and can show up in the first year. Boys are slower to pick up language, so be less concerned if, say, young Billy isn't keeping up with his sister's pace or if some of the boys in the class have trouble keeping up with some of the fast-talking precocious girls. However, a parent should become concerned with boys *and* girls as a child approaches his or her first birthday if some of the following signals are detected.

Signals

- The child is selective in what he hears, "ignoring" many directives.
- Some questions are understood, while others don't get through.
- A parent or caregiver must repeat him- or herself several times, or begins to speak more slowly and in a louder tone of voice.
- Simple instructions don't seem to be comprehended and certainly are not followed.
- The child doesn't pick up on ordinary conversation starters— "Eat?" "Let's clap!" "Daddy says hi."

Usual Misinterpretations

- Parents often confuse difficulty with receptive language processing as being a sign of stubbornness or of a child who pays attention only to what interests her.
- In many cases, parents and pediatricians wonder about a child's hearing.
- Parents, teachers, and caregivers often confuse slowness in language receptivity to be sure signs of either future learning problems or even retardation. The labels have the implication that a child is "slow." Though there is some evidence that late talkers do have a greater chance of developing learning difficulties, this is by no means an accurate indicator of intelligence.

Questions to Ask (Parents, Caregivers, Pediatricians, Teachers)

- When did her "hearing" problem start?
- Does he always ignore you?
- Does it make a difference to speak more slowly?
- When she can see your face, does she respond more easily?
- Do you find yourself raising your voice, or generally speaking louder to get his attention?

Where to Refer

If there is little improvement within the first year, hearing *should* be checked first. And if speech doesn't begin to come in, a speech and language pathologist needs to be contacted. Evaluations are now possible at very early ages. Find a childhood developmental team (usually such groups are connected to large hospitals or child agencies) who specialize in our youngest children.

Disturbances in Expressive Language

Expressive language is the ability to speak, articulate, and organize language—to initiate and respond to simple conversation.

Signals

- Late onset of speech. There is a real gender difference here. Most language specialists become concerned about boys, whose speech tends to develop later, somewhere between 2 and 3 years old. With girls, one begins to notice problems at around 2 years of age.
- Echolalia. While most early language is largely imitative, echolalia has a different feel. It is the repetitive matching of phrases and words that a child hears. Children who exhibit echolalia may repeat words they've heard literally hundreds of times. For example, "How are you doing?" regularly will be met with "How you doing?" rather than "Hi, Mommy."
- Word retrieval. While telling a story, the child can't find the right word or words. He takes a long time searching and is obviously having difficulty expressing what he means to say.
- High frustration level. Kids who have trouble with expressive language often get frustrated easily. They can't find the words, have trouble organizing coherent sentences, and because of this naturally get very mad when words fail.
- Organization. It is normal, of course, for young children's sentences to be disorganized and for stories to ramble on and be jumbled up. But for children who have trouble with expressive language, organization almost always is missing a beginning, middle, or end. This is a later development, and shouldn't be of concern until the third or fourth year.
- "Language pragmatics." This means speech isn't used to further social relationships or get needs met: a child grabs instead of asking, can't negotiate games with other kids.

Usual Misinterpretations

- Parents tend to put off evaluation, because living with a child every day one gets used to speech peculiarities.
- "It's just a phase," parents and teachers think, "She'll talk when she's ready."

- It's manipulative: "He has everyone reading his mind."
- Often problems with expressive language are confused with personality types: "She's shy." "He's a loner." "She's never been a big conversationalist."

Questions to Ask

- When did your child first start to talk?
- Did he begin gradually or start with complete sentences?
- Does she compulsively repeat words or phrases?
- Does he have trouble finding the right words?
- Does she easily get words mixed up?
- Does he have trouble with words like prepositions that describe direction—often getting them backward: on–off, above–below, before–after?
- Does she use language to get what she wants in social relationships?
- Is it a problem in articulation (which means clarity of pronunciation)? Articulation is often simply mechanical—moving lips, tongue properly versus a problem in language processing.
- Does the child get very angry not being able to express himself?
- Do other children the child's age have trouble understanding what she says or being able to play games in a cooperative way?

Where to Refer

If any of these signals continue with boys and girls until 2½, calling in a speech and language specialist is a must. He or she will do a simple and nontraumatic evaluation and can begin to establish whether there is indeed a problem. If needed, methods of intervention are easy to apply, and can be used by both language specialists and parents at home. Early speech intervention has been shown to make an enormous difference in a child's future language development.

Relatedness

The second area affected by PDD that is often extremely apparent to the helping professional is loosely called "relatedness." This has to do with the basic level of relationship, connection, and bonding that a child is capable of. Professionals and parents should pay attention to the following:

Signals

- Early bonding with mother or primary caretaker did not come easily. Parents describe various ways in which a good connection was not made: poor feeding habits, difficulty "molding" to Mom's body, or problems becoming settled. This is not to be confused with the first few months of unsettled behavior that most babies go through, especially difficult or colicky children. Rather, a slowness to connect to even primary caretakers continues through the first year of life.
- Mothers will describe a lack of satisfaction in bonding, less back-and-forth exchanges.
- As the child gets older, she shows less interest in peers than other kids.
- The child prefers to play alone, often engaging in repetitive behaviors.
- The child tends to wander off alone in social settings.
- One observes less stranger anxiety at the usual age, which is approximately 8 months. The child is not afraid of strangers, and yet he is not drawn into making new friends.
- As the child enters preschool and day care, her mother reports that she is not sought out for play dates with other kids.

Delays in two other areas of development also become apparent within the first few years of life: (1) *gross and fine motor development*; (2) *feeding difficulties*. They may not seem to be part of "relatedness" but are sometimes indications of PDD and significantly affect a child's ability to make connections with others.

Gross and Fine Motor Coordination

Kids along the PDD continuum often have difficulty in areas of gross motor coordination that affect their capacity to play:

- Difficulties with what is called "crossing the midline of one's body." This means that it is hard for the child to move her left hand over toward the right side of her body and visa versa. Midline difficulties are manifested by a propensity for PDD kids to build *upward*. Blocks and Legos, for example, are stacked vertically, rather than outward.
- Children in this category often sit on the floor with legs crossed not in yoga position but with legs angled backward in the shape of a "W."
- Some children also engage in what is called "toe-walking." They prefer walking on either the balls or toes of their feet.
- Kids have difficulty with fine motor skills that are part of daily life—tying shoe laces; they may also have trouble developing other skill areas—block building, drawing, or writing letters.
- "Low-tone" kids. Some of these children may have less muscle strength, usually in the upper body. This inhibits ability to engage in the usual roughhousing, or games requiring physical exertion.

Usual Misinterpretations

The usual misinterpretation is that it is all physical (which should be checked out, as there may be some delay in muscular development):

- If a boy or girl only builds in a masculine/phallic manner, it is misinterpreted as an indicator of underlying gender issues.
- Difficulties with fine motor skills can be viewed, in girls, as also gender related—"They're like boys."
- A boy who displays low tone or lack of aptitude in gross motor skills is often labeled by adults and peers as being a "sissy" or "spastic."

Feeding Difficulties

This area is probably the least understood by helping professionals yet has enormous consequences on relatedness to caregivers and sense of parents' self-worth. Feeding difficulties are also indicators of developmental delays and occasionally PDD. Yet, because so much is culturally associated with food, parents explain away important signals of underlying treatable disorders with euphemisms such as "finicky," "bad eater," or "insatiable." Feeding difficulties manifest themselves in many subtle ways and need to be taken especially seriously when certain signals are apparent from the earliest days of life or are severe. They usually become apparent after the introduction of solid foods and include the following:

- The texture of certain foods are uncomfortable for the child to touch. They feel too greasy, juicy, slimy, or wet.
- A kid will only tolerate a narrow range of food. Those that are too spicy or have strong smells can be very disturbing to him.
- A child may often be a slow eater. Food seems boring, especially when compared to her siblings or peers.
- The child doesn't show the usual enthusiasm for "treats" at parties.
- He won't sit at the dinner table for too long.
- She tends to wander around and become extremely distracted in restaurants.
- Some kids are put off, even repulsed, by seeing others eat.

Usual Misinterpretations

What makes this area so difficult for both child and parents is that it is especially open to misinterpretation. Unaware parents and even skilled professionals may view an eating difficulty as a power struggle, or defiance. Mothers, in particular, feel very discouraged, upset that they are being personally rejected. Distraction, trickery, and coaxing are used to get more food accepted by the child, which then *does* potentially lead to serious power struggles. It is much more effective to find out whether the child has a primary feeding difficulty and refer him to a specialist.

Questions to Ask

- Has the child always been uninterested in food?
- Will he eat *some* foods?
- What type, texture, color?
- How much at a time?
- Is she a "grazer" or does she "gulp" it down?
- Was he a better eater and then suddenly stopped?
- Have there been any big changes in the household recently?
- Does she like small portions?
- Is he fussy about changes in eating routines?
- Does she eat differently at other people's houses?

Where to Refer

If there is a pattern of general difficulty with food, present from the time of nursing or with the introduction of solid foods, the child should be referred to either a feeding specialist (these specialists are still hard to find but will, I predict, become numerous during the next 5 years) or an occupational therapist (these professionals are in fact becoming very much in demand in all major urban and suburban areas). A diagnosis can be made as to whether eating problems are a manifestation of sensory defensiveness (described below) or whether there is a medical, environmental, or behavioral reason for the difficulty.

Sensory Defensiveness

Sensory defensiveness is one of the least recognized and yet one of the most recent and important areas discovered in child development. It explains a multitude of unusual behaviors in children and is often the third indicator of PDD. Keep in mind that many children, like those with feeding difficulties, have some aspects of sensory defensiveness. Without delays in language development or difficulties in relatedness, PDD is not usually an appropriate diagnosis.

Basically, sensory defensiveness has to do with a child's ability to take in and comfortably integrate stimuli. The human body has numerous sensory systems: sight, sound, taste, smell, tactile, kinesthetic, among others. Children who have varying degrees of sensory defensiveness are uncomfortable dealing with or taking in one or more of these stimuli. This discomfort gets in the way of dealing with new situations, relating to other children, and functioning in school. Here are some of the most typical manifestations:

Signals

- Gaze aversion. Making eye contact with another person, even with Mom, feels uncomfortable to a child and he averts his eyes. Gaze aversion is particularly apparent with adults outside the family, with peers, and especially with strangers.
- Fabric sensitivity. Many parents can relate to this form of sensory defensiveness. Children are extremely uncomfortable wearing scratchy clothing, labels, specific kinds of material. With some, seams are problematic, as is tight, binding clothing.
- Mess. Children who are sensory defensive will cry about dirty diapers and don't like to touch messy play materials such as Play Doh. They have a great deal of difficulty with finger painting.
- There is discomfort walking on rough surfaces, such as grass, sand, and pebbly beaches.
- Light touch. This is another area of tactile discomfort in which kids, much to their parents' dismay, don't like being stroked gently.
- Lights and noises. Many of these children have trouble in big screen movie theaters that are visually and auditorally intense. They avoid uncomfortable sounds by covering their ears, sounds that would not seem particularly loud to most

people. Sudden noises can be frightening: fireworks, concerts, or large stadiums are a veritable nightmare.

Usual Misinterpretations

Depending on the area of a child's sensory defensiveness, different interpretations are typical. Kids who hold their hands over their ears are thought to be antisocial; children who refuse to wear anything but a narrow range of clothing are labeled overly sensitive or spoiled, like *The Princess and the Pea*. As kids get older, mothers feel manipulated and bossed around by their demanding, seemingly fussy children.

Generally, the area of sensory defensiveness is one of the most widespread yet undiagnosed syndromes from which children suffer. What is most disturbing is that unless addressed, labels, power struggles, and pejorative interpretations follow, which unfortunately, over time, can easily become self-fulfilling prophesies.

Questions to Ask

The questions to ask for sensory defensiveness are obvious. They have to do with finding out whether a child has always had an oversensitivity in any of the areas described above.

Where to Refer

When a teacher, pediatrician, or parent spots any of these signals, it's extremely helpful to ask for an evaluation by an occupational therapist (OT). Every professional who works with children should, in my opinion, have an OT on their team. This specialist can evaluate and offer specific interventions for the child. Interventions consist of gradually desensitizing kids to whichever stimuli cause the most trouble. For example, a child who has difficulty getting "messy" is introduced to increasingly more uncomfortable play materials. Eventually, a child's system becomes less reactive. Kids can then slowly be involved in activities that had once been too uncomfortable to even go near.

Obsessive–Compulsive and Anxiety Disorders

Most professionals who work with children think of obsessive–compulsive disorder (OCD) in its much more grown-up manifestations—obsessional hand washing, checking, and the like. But in children who have are predisposed to OCD, the signals are much more subtle. There are two types of OCD: one type exists in the world of action; the other, in the world of thinking. However, both have a similar feel to parents and professionals: "The needle gets stuck on the record." And both types are vulnerable to panic and anxiety attacks.

OCD in the Area of Behavior

Signals

- A child needs to have rituals and routines that cannot be altered in any way. If the normal bedtime procedure is changed, or the route walking to school needs to be adjusted for some reason, or foods are served in a different order, then anger, rather than anxiety, is the typical reaction.
- Kids have trouble playing the usual fantasy and make-believe games of childhood. His inclinations are more concrete, preferring activities that are repetitive and mechanical.
- Transitions are particularly difficult. A child gets stuck, becoming extremely agitated and angry when a parent attempts to move things along.

Usual Misinterpretations

- These children often are interpreted as being extremely stubborn, even tyrannical, self-centered, and shallow.
- Behavior is normalized. Because it is so much a part of everyday life—"just her way"—parents don't even notice idiosyncrasies.
- Parents mold themselves to their kids' unusual demands,

thinking their child to be "high strung," and so avoid any chance for an explosion.

Questions to Ask

- Do you feel as if you're walking on eggshells?
- Do your child's reactions scare you?
- How often does this happen—once a day, once a week?
- How long does your child stay angry and anxious?
- Can he be soothed by hugging or talking?
- Can she only be soothed by giving her what she demands?
- Does he prefer his routines more than playing with other kids?

OCD in the Area of Thought

When OCD affects thinking, kids are ruminative worriers, prone to anxiety attacks. Just like children with behavior compulsions, they are experienced by parents as youngsters whose needles get stuck. Only with these kids, parents become extremely frustrated, as well as occasionally scared. If one worry after the other pops up, panic lurks in the shadows. Worries are as varied as one's imagination but usually include the following:

- Fears about the night and death
- Hypochondriacal concerns for oneself and significant others
- Separation anxiety and worry about losing parents
- Body image concerns in younger children and boys
- Preoccupation and fascination with public tragedies, natural disasters, and the like.

Signals

There are several ways to distinguish obsessional worry from normal childhood fears:

- Frequency. Normal childhood fears are occasionally triggered by changes in development or in life circumstances. Obsessional worries seem to "come out of nowhere" and occur several times a month, a week, or even a day.

- Intensity. Normal childhood fears can often be soothed by holding, talking, or a little bit of extra attention. Obsessional worries, on the other hand, are not responsive to discussion or other soothing behaviors; they just seem to run their course.
- When normal childhood fears scare most kids, they often worry about becoming frightened again; but when an obsessional worry is over for a child with OCD, " it seems as if it never happened." The child has forgotten about what had been previously of paramount importance—until the next worry appears.
- Normal fears elicit sympathy in parents; obsessional worries, because of their intransigent nature, elicit parents' frustration and anger.
- The "rain-barrel" effect. After a number of ruminative worries accumulate, anxiety and panic attacks can follow.

Usual Misinterpretations

- The child is doing it on purpose.
- He is insatiably needy or clingy.
- She is being argumentative, just to be difficult.
- They're not genuine needs, but rather are being used manipulatively to get extra attention.

Questions to Ask

- How often does the child have such worry attacks?
- Can she be soothed and, if so, how?
- In the midst of an obsession, does he seem to be in almost a trance-like state, unavailable to rational argument or advice?
- Does it affect her ongoing mood and continue as a quiet preoccupation in the background?
- Is the worry strong enough to get in the way of playing and having fun?

Where to Refer

There are two routes to go. The first is to a cognitive-behavioral therapist. He or she will work with a child using strategies that have been proven quite effective in diminishing compulsive behavior and obsessional thinking. The second avenue is a pharmacological evaluation by a child psychiatrist, especially if there have been panic attacks. Extremely small amounts of serotonin stimulators— Prozac, Zoloft, etc.—along with behaviorally oriented treatment, are often astonishingly helpful. With the constellation of OCD symptoms, nondirective play therapy is not, in my experience, effective. If anything, these modalities don't reduce obsessional thinking and compulsive behaviors; in fact, they may become even worse. Talk therapy, individual and family, *is* helpful, however, with anxiety disorders. Although still controversial, I've found that brief courses of medication are also needed.

Childhood Depression

Childhood depression is quite different from adult depression in that kids' moods are much more fluid. Even depressed children can lose themselves in activities and appear to be perfectly OK. This is why it is particularly important that the adults in a child's life understand the subtle signals of childhood depression. They are the following:

Signals

- Negative evaluations by the child about her experiences. These almost always make an event the child's fault or a result of her own inadequacy. "The soccer game was lost because of me," or "Nobody in the group likes me, because of the way I look."
- Depressed children are often highly self-aware to the point of being painfully self-conscious. It is hard to let go without being at least a little self-aware. It is as if they are watching themselves having fun.

- Kids often relate better to older folks or very young children. "Old before their time" is a phrase that seems to fit such kids.
- Some depressed children, far from giving up on life, do just the opposite: they try too hard, become too serious, and are overly concerned about how well they are doing in school or sports.

Usual Misinterpretations

- "They're just being good children" or "Our best little girl or boy in the world."
- They are seen as "weak"—overly compliant and cooperative to a fault.
- Caretaker kids, they seem "gifted" in their ability to empathize with the feelings of others, especially the elderly, infirm, or disadvantaged.
- They are labeled uptight and repeatedly encouraged to just loosen up.

Questions to Ask

- How long have you noticed this in your child?
- Was there a change in your family or life circumstances?
- Does he ever see the glass as half full?
- Does she seem compelled to take care of friends who are unhappy?
- Does he open up about what's bothering him?
- Are you afraid of saying the wrong things?
- Does she stand up for herself with other kids?
- Do you often feel like you want to help, fix things, or cheer him up?

Where to Refer

Again, cognitive therapy is particularly effective with long-standing pessimism and mild to moderate childhood depression. If a child does not respond to such non-medical intervention, it is important to refer for a pharmacological evaluation. This is especially so if a child talks about "running away," "being a burden," or makes any comments about "life not being worth it."

Depressive Reaction

There are many children who do not exhibit long-standing pessimistic or depressive attitudes. However, in response to developmental changes or traumatic life circumstances, they can have fairly severe depressive reactions. This mood change is apparent to almost everyone, but here is the often paralyzing dilemma: Should we do anything, or is this just a phase that will pass? Here are some ways to make a distinction.

Signals

- A phase lifts within weeks. A depressive reaction will continue on for several months, if not longer.
- A phase is not so all-encompassing. Even in the midst of it, hours and days can pass without any disturbance in mood. A true depressive reaction, while rarely continuous, affects most aspects of a child's daily life.
- Depressive reactions effect a child's vegetative/physiological functions (i.e., his appetite for food and sleep–wake cycles). Because of this, there is often either a gain or a loss of weight.
- Children ignore their usual passions. If interests remain, lower endurance is noticeable, as well as less ability to focus on activities.
- Depressive reactions usually predispose kids to be easily thrown by transitions during the day. Before, transitions had not presented much of a problem.

Usual Misinterpretations

- It is a "phase" that will pass without adult intervention.
- The child is being overly sensitive and should just "toughen up."

- It is somebody else's fault—a bad teacher, caregiver, classroom placement (which may be true, and should be explored).

Generally speaking, whatever a child's weakest link in his personality, this is where his depressive symptom will be most apparent. So, if a child is prone to fears, he will be more fearful; if he is normally clingy and has difficulty at bedtime, he will become even harder to put down.

Questions to Ask

- What has recently changed in the environment?
- How have you tried to adapt to the new situation?
- Has this affected his sleep, appetite, or usual interests?
- Can she "forget" about it and play with friends?
- Does he talk about leaving, or running away?
- Is there someone she talks to in the family?

Where to Refer

If there are strong family supports, medication is usually not needed. If the depressive mood continues, referrals should be made to short-term, individual and family therapy. The child can talk about his feelings in individual treatment; at the same time, family sessions are useful to problem-solve and air emotions. A medication evaluation should be considered if you are concerned about the child's safety or if other interventions do not help.

Attention Deficit Disorder

Popular sentiment has it that attention deficit disorder (ADD) and attention-deficit/hyperactivity disorder (ADHD) are the diagnoses of the moment and are used far too frequently. My experience is exactly the opposite. Because most people, including professionals who work with children, view ADD in a rather narrow and linear fashion, in my opinion it is actually *under*diagnosed. The problem, I believe, is one of definition. ADD does not mean total inability to focus, nor does it mean (and most professionals *do* understand this) the presence of hyperactivity. ADD is not a black or white concept; rather, it exists along a continuum, in a much less formal fashion—problems in focusing take different shapes and forms—and indirectly affect many aspects of a child's functioning.

This wider definition has paid off in dramatic fashion. Many kids who had been previously limping along in their lives, just barely passing in school, and marginal with their peers, make significant changes when the following more subtle signals of ADD are recognized and treated. They are:

Signals

- An inability to self-reflect. Children with ADD are often impulsive. So are many other kids. What distinguishes ADD impulsivity from other types is that afterward kids with ADD have absolutely no idea why they did what they did— no plan, no apparent motivation: "It just happened."
- Low threshold for boredom. Kids with ADD are so averse to boredom they will do almost anything—clown around, start a fight with a sibling, act out impulsively—just to avoid feeling bored.
- Kids with ADD are often incredibly defensive and quick to come up with explanations as to why it's somebody else's fault. This glib dissembling turns into outright lying if ADD is not picked up on.
- Kids with ADD have explosive, angry outbursts. This is particularly so when frustrated about not getting something. What throws most parents and professionals off is the level of focus kids with ADD are capable of—when it comes to something they want. This is especially apparent over "the

stuff." By this I mean the gear that is constantly advertised in the media.

- Kids with ADD are insatiable pop culture addicts, can watch TV or play video games endlessly without getting bored. This is quite different from most kids who also love TV but after a couple of hours become restless. Kids with ADD seem to calm down and almost go into an altered state. TV becomes a companion to such kids. As one articulate adolescent boy put it, "I feel like television creates a nice, soft container around me." Most kids with ADD will instantly turn on TV the moment they enter the house.
- Kids with ADD get into clumsy accidents and are seen as accident prone.
- Kids with ADD are into "future-wanting." This means that there's always something new on the horizon that must be gotten: new toys, new movies, product tie-ins are always on these kids' minds. Future-wanting becomes the center of their lives.
- The outbursts of kids with ADD are not like the tantrums we see in other children; rather, they are exceptionally focused. It is as if the anger helps organize such a child's usual distracted inner experience.
- Kids with ADD daydream almost continuously when no outside interesting stimulation is available. This is especially so with girls for whom acting out and hyperactivity is not as socially acceptable and because fantasy games are a central part of normal girls' psychic development.

Usual Misinterpretations

Many parents believe that these kids don't care, are selfish, and are entirely unmotivated. They are often viewed as being less intelligent or simply not "school types." Learning difficulties may be picked up in school, such as problems in reading or in math. But the accompanying attentional difficulty is all too often ignored. Finally, numbers of progressive-minded adults attribute attentional weakness to a problem with self-confidence or anxiety about trying new things.

Questions to Ask

The questions that help a professional can be adapted from all of the points made above on pages 39 to 40.

Where to Refer

If you find the signals I just described, a referral needs to be immediately made. Problems with attention do not disappear over time, nor will traditional talk, play, or family therapy address it in a satisfactory manner. In the same way, psychological testing, which many people incorrectly believe can diagnose ADD, is not terribly effective in detecting this syndrome.

The first course of action is an educational battery (to find underlying learning disabilities). Teachers should fill out behavioral questionnaires such as the Conners Scale, and—this is *crucial*—a psychiatric evaluation should be done by a doctor who *specializes* in ADD. It is important to send a child and family to someone who has a lot of expertise picking up on the subtle cues of attentional disorders. In my experience, too often no diagnosis is made and no subsequent action is taken.

Summary Checklist

Once you become aware of what the problems are, the subtle signals of ADD are, in fact, extremely apparent. Within minutes of your asking a child about his interests, problems with attention will come to your mind. As you will see, almost all ADD pursuits have the following characteristics:

- They are done with other kids.
- Adults are not necessary.
- There are few strict rules and guidelines.
- They are outside the mainstream of school, sports, and organized activities.

- They are self-regulated and require little delay of gratification and instruction.

When you hear about heavy involvement in the following interests, begin to think about attentional or learning problems:

- In-line skating
- Snowboarding
- Skateboarding
- Cult magazines
- Fantasy video games—especially violent products
- Alternative comic books: in particular X-rated, violence-saturated ones
- Identifying with the "slacker" group in school
- Intense preoccupation with clothes, style, and makeup along with little academic motivation
- Marijuana as the drug of choice
- Cravings for caffeinated foods, which sometimes help *calm* a child—chocolate, diet sodas, coffee, etc.

Of course, many kids in a our culture today are drawn to these tastes and interests. Keep in mind, though, that what distinguishes children who may have underlying attentional problems is an almost total absence of any pursuit that requires adult presence, practice, or delay of gratification.

*   *   *

Remember, this is not meant to be an official diagnostic manual. There are other conditions, such as Asperger's and Tourette's syndromes, that are relatively rare which I have not included. Check the *Diagnostic and Statistical Manual of Mental Disorders, 4th edition* (DSM-IV, 1994) or the *Zero–Three Diagnostic Guide* (National Center for Clinical Infant Programs, 1994) for more information.

However, I *have* included many of the most common and yet least recognized difficulties. Follow these hands-on guidelines and you will save many kids and parents from often unnecessary suffering. Spotting problems also helps other group members: a correctly treated child can, as I've observed many times, settle down an entire classroom; groups of kids at camp or in an after-school activity are able to become more involved when they are not distracted by a child who is disruptive. When you see these symptoms and signs, it is time to suggest consultation with a specialist if you cannot offer expert advice.

Remember, as I learned in my interviews with children, kids want and need adults in their lives who know what's going on. Learning to correctly understand when a child requires help is one way of providing this leadership.

chapter three

Tough Tykes

Getting Through to Difficult Children
(2–10 Years Old)

For some kids, their basic temperamental characteristics seem to stand in the way of change. These kids often get labeled "difficult." While knowing diagnostic categories is important (such as the diagnoses ADD, ADHD, OCD, and childhood depression, which I cover in Chapter 2), children with difficult temperaments often fall between the cracks. Their behaviors are tough to budge, yet they're not serious enough to be diagnosable.

The area of temperament, while discovered decades ago by Alexander Thomas and Stella Chess (*Temperament and Behavior Disorders in Children*, New York University Press, 1968), was virtually ignored in mainstream work with children until the mid-1990s. It remains one of the last frontiers. Most professionals working with kids are just remotely familiar with it as a concept. Temperament is the constellation of attributes that a child comes into the world with. It is not *caused* by parent error. Temperament can be described as how a child is different "in nature" from his siblings or friends—and has been different in these ways from the time he was born. Clinical studies about temperament are revolutionizing the way we look at kids and also putting into perspective how much a child's personality impacts on family life.

When parents approach us many believe a child is bad or *they* are entirely to blame for a child's difficult behavior. Professionals who know the half dozen main characteristics of temperament are able to help parents more fully understand their child without negatively judging themselves. A profound message can be imparted:

- "I know what you have to deal with."
- "You did not create her personality."
- "I understand what causes your child to act this way."
- "Together we can make things better."

I cannot describe the gratitude parents feel when someone finally grasps the impact of temperament. So, to add an understanding of temperament to your approach with parents and kids, I include below the six major traits that I have found the most helpful in understanding how kids experience their world.

Each trait includes the colloquial phrases parents use to describe a child. These can serve as red flags of how temperamental factors may contribute to a difficult situation. I've also added typical ways mothers and fathers misinterpret a child and blame themselves. These misinterpretations are a major source of unhappiness parents experience, even when they seek our help.

The Six Major Characteristics of Temperament

1. Initial Reaction to New Experiences

Description

Children have different inborn ways they respond to new experiences. This is called *initial reaction*. Simply put, it refers to how a child deals with unfamiliar situations. For example, some kids are not as gregarious as their parents would like. They hang at the edge of groups. They are shy and don't immediately move into the center of the action. Andrea, the parent of such a child, misunderstood this initial hesitation, interpreting it as defiance on the part of 4-

year-old Ethan. "He doesn't want to listen to me. He doesn't respect that I am his mother." In fact, a brief developmental history showed that Ethan always had problems with initial reaction.

My own children are quite different in how they react to new situations. One of my kids, Sammy, doesn't take well to new people, appearing at first to be antisocial. It takes him quite a while to work his way into a group. Our other child, Leah, is quite gregarious, and moves into many new settings without a moment's hesitation. It made a tremendous difference for my wife and myself to "get" that this was not our fault, rather the way each of our children were born.

Misinterpretations

A parent might say about his or her child:

> "He's too shy."
> "She's a scaredy cat."
> "He's afraid to take risks."
> "She seems to be antisocial."

A parent might say about him- or herself:

> "I push too hard."
> "I didn't push hard enough."
> "Have I done things to scare my own child?"

2. Adaptability

Description

Some kids are flexible. They can tolerate being whisked from one activity to the next. Their disposition is resilient enough to adjust to the changes and variations many transitions demand. This is unlike 6-year-old Dom, who can only tolerate one major activity a day. Any more, and Dom's parents take the risk of his experiencing a meltdown. Or the mother of 4-year-old Peter came in and reported, "I don't know what to do. My son doesn't want to leave the house. When we need to go somewhere he balks, and he doesn't listen to our directions. It drives us crazy." Peter has greater difficulty than other children dealing with transitions, and what his parents are describing is, again, an inborn discomfort adapting to various situations. Obviously, children with less adaptability suffer more during times of major transition—divorce, sickness, or family relocation. Eight-year-old George was such a child. He exhibited the classic behaviors of a youngster who has trouble adapting. After his father's job relocation and the family's subsequent move, George regressed in many of his ordinary behaviors. He had trouble getting down to bed at night, and just wanted to watch TV rather than venture out and play in his wonderful backyard.

Misinterpretations

A parent might say about his or her child:

> "He needs his routine."
> "She's rigid and bossy."
> "He has no flexibility."
> "She flips out when she doesn't get her way."
> "We need to build our lives around his schedule."
> "How come other parents can take their kids anywhere?"

A parent might say about him- or herself:

> "What did I do to raise such a rigid kid?"
> "I don't know how to manage the day's activities right."
> "There must be something wrong with my tone, or the way I speak with him."

Activity Level

Description

The next characteristic is one we're all familiar with: activity level. There are a vast number of kids not diagnosable with ADD, yet they simply wear a parent down. They are almost always on the move. Many parents would, in fact, define activity level as one of the key characteristics of a child being easy or difficult. For example, at a party most of the kids were climbing the walls. One child, Lowell, however, sat on his mom's lap almost the entire time. Lowell is a child who is developmentally normal in every way; he just has a lower activity level and was described by envious parents as being an "easy" kid. Most parents who approach us are not as lucky as Lowell's. It is important to be able to distinguish between a child with a high activity level and one with ADHD (see the accompanying box).

Misinterpretations

Activity level varies tremendously between kids and is again easily misinterpreted by parents as being a child-rearing failure, rather

---

Distinguishing between Highly Active Children and Children with ADHD

OVERLY ACTIVE CHILDREN	CHILDREN WITH ADHD
Happiest when they're moving about	Rarely, if ever, let up
Can settle down for longer periods of time	Maintain a breakneck pace throughout the day
Have few reports of aggressive outbursts towards other kids or siblings	As a rule, are more aggressive and prone to rages
Go through different times of the day that are better or worse	Are predisposed to impulsive behaviors throughout the day
Can reflect and talk about behaviors afterward	Have a difficult, if not impossible, time reflecting about behaviors afterward

than an inborn characteristic usually having roots in one's family history.

A parent might say about his or her child:

"He's wearing me down."
"I never get to relax for a minute."
"It's like living with a tornado."
"She was always an active child."
"He was even like this while I carried him."

A parent might say about him- or herself:

"She must be picking the tension up in our house."
"I don't know how to be a soothing presence."
"I don't have the energy to be a parent."
"I can't stand having children."

Tenacity

Description

Some kids are born with the ability to "lock" onto something. No amount of distraction gets such children to let go of what they've set their sights on. This tunnel vision can be about food, a material item such as a toy, or even an idea—a play date scheduled for the end of the day. Recently, I was talking to a strong-willed teenager, Nadine, who describes herself as always "wanting what I want." Nadine can remember being driven since she was 4 years old. Even if a parent is philosophically and morally against corporal punishment, kids who are very tenacious often provoke a physical response in their parents.

Muriel is the mother of 5-year-old Ina. She was distraught because Ina seemed so relentless and determined to get what she wanted. This quiet, gentle human being often felt like grabbing her daughter and shaking some sense into her. Tenacious kids also seem immune to typical discipline techniques. This is what Alex told me about his son, David: "Negative consequences don't work. We've taken everything away from him already. Just yesterday, David said 'Go ahead. I don't care what you do. Punish me, but I still want to get that Gameboy.' " The ante with these kids always seems to be escalating, with parents repeatedly at the edge of losing control.

Misinterpretations

A parent might say about his or her child:

> "She's like a bull."
> "He's always thinking one step ahead."
> "I feel like I'm constantly negotiating."
> "She seems to be tougher than me."
> "My child is evil in how manipulative he can become."

A parent might say about him- or herself:

> "She's inherited my worst characteristics."
> "I'm a doormat."
> "It's because my spouse and I don't agree."
> "I'm not consistent enough."

Sensitivity

Description

Immortalized by *The Princess and the Pea*, these children are painfully sensitive to many types of stimulation. At one end of this continuum is a child such as Sophie, who has trouble when the classroom is too loud or when she goes to a large screen movie or to see fireworks. Another sensitive child, Alan, has trouble with coarse clothing or slimy kinds of activities like finger painting.

At the other end of the continuum are children whose sensitivity to stimulation is so strong they are what we call "sensory defensive" (see p. 29 for more details). This is a need to block out different kinds of sensory input at many levels: sight, sound, smell, fabric, food texture, extreme temperatures, and even internal emotions. Parents of such children in particular feel as if they are walking on eggshells. Worse, they often feel extremely rejected—kids who are sensory defensive often have trouble making eye contact or responding to tactile affection, such as light stroking or hugs.

Such was the case with Samara. Meeting her parents was quite an ordeal. They had gotten used to an enormous range of Samara's special needs: soft clothing, foods that were crunchy and dry, and her aversion to loud noises in nursery school and to the sights and sounds of big movies. Samara's parents knew something wasn't right. She was slightly different from other kids, but they didn't know why or how. Dad blamed Mom for giving in and spoiling Samara, but Mom had a deep sense, during those few moments she was not angrily defensive, that something wasn't quite right.

Misinterpretations

What a parent might say about his or her child:

"My child is a crybaby."
"He's so particular about everything."
"She's such a finicky person."
"The world revolves around him."

What a parent might say about him- or herself:

"How did we spoil her so much?"
"Will I ever be able to prepare him to live in the world?"
"We should never have picked her up so much."
"She's got her father completely twisted around her finger."

Mood

Description

Mood combines a lot of different elements: optimism versus pessimism; outgoing versus reserved. In short, some kids are simply more upbeat and resilient, evidencing a wonderful, infectious mood. "Life is a bowl of cherries," they seem to say, even as babies. Of course, they have their moments and go through temporary "down" phases, but they're resilient and the glass seems perpetually to be half full. They are not sensitive; they adapt to new situations; they don't have trouble with initial reactions or with other kids.

On the other hand, some kids are simply less effusive. Not troublemakers, they blend in and, though nobody notices much, their light seems to burn a little less brightly. In group situations, they do well. Play, school routines, and structured activities bring out the best in them. But at home parents see a less enthusiastic camper. They seem, as Chloe described Jessica, her youngest daughter, to be almost petulant. Jessica, like many other kids prone to moodiness, often needs an adult around for affection and company. Such children's endurance seems to be lower, and their tenacity as compared to some of the children described above is much less fierce.

Parents whose children have less exuberant moods are often the most critical of themselves and terribly confused about what is going on. The world tells them that everything is OK, and their worries are those of the overanxious mother. For example, Maria, mother of a 4-year-old, low-keyed Becky, could always sense her daughter's potential lower moods, but in public Becky would participate well enough. And in structured activities she became involved and really had a good time.

Once Becky got home, though, Mom and Dad would see another side. Here's where her petulance and low threshold for disappointment and fatigue would be more apparent. As Maria described so poignantly, "Why is it that she's acted so normally in school, yet seems to be so hard to please and even moody at home?"

Mothers, especially, blame themselves when they have a child with a slightly less exuberant mood. They worry about early deprivation, believe that some secret trauma may have happened to their child, that they made some terrible mistakes about feeding, toilet training, or amount of the time spent together. Of course, all of these are possible. But I have found that the more likely explanation is temperament. A child's mood, if stable from the earliest years, is not anyone's fault; it's simply part of her natural endowment.

Misinterpretations

What a parent might say about a child:

"She's so dependent."
"Things seem to quickly make him unhappy."
"A bad mood always seems to be just around the corner."
"As soon as there's a break in the action, she gets kind of sullen."
"He's lazy—she doesn't seem to have too many great interests, such as hobbies or after-school activities."
"How did I fail her early in life?"
"Did I not give him a happy enough foundation?"
"Did some kind of bad experience happen with babysitters or other people that I don't know about?"
"Is there something physically the matter?"

What to Do with Difficult Children

Drawing a "Tempogram"

To help a parent become more optimistic and compassionate about a difficult child, draw what I call a "tempogram." This is a visual aid that shows a parent how different aspects of temperament run through the family and can't simply be a creation of bad parenting. A tempogram is really a family tree that focuses on the temperamental characteristic most apparent and troublesome in a child's behavior. It includes the parents' children, their own siblings, and their parents (see the accompanying figure). For example, Pauline approached the teacher of her first grader, Scott, complaining how bullheaded he was. "What had she done wrong to create such a tyrant?" she wondered, indirectly implying

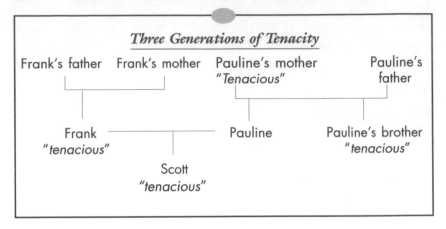

that the teacher was somehow also at fault. The teacher, Elaine, consulted me and with my encouragement asked Pauline several "tempogram" questions, such as "Is there anyone else in your family who has been tenacious or bullheaded like Scott?" Within a couple of minutes of polite conversation, they realized that Scott had been tenacious from the get-go and was not unlike Elaine's brother and her husband's mother.

This brief exercise immediately reduced blame and bewilderment. It increased Pauline's compassion for herself and, most important, diminished the unrealistic hope that one day Pauline would wake up and Scott would suddenly be less of a formidable character to deal with.

Specific Recommendations for Specific Temperaments

The Zero to Three Foundation, along with other research centers around the country, have recommended ways to handle children who have different temperamental characteristics. I've synthesized their findings with my own. This brief guide is helpful in encouraging parents to be more effective with difficult children. It is also extremely valuable in helping teachers, guidance counselors, as well as therapists offer more specific feedback to parents (see the accompanying box on page 55).

Summary: Distinguishing Temperamental Characteristics from "Bad Parenting"

Several questions are helpful to make the distinction. Be sure to ask parents:

1. How long have they noticed this characteristic?
2. Since first year of life? . . . earlier?
3. Any others in family history you've heard about?
4. Have you always had a sense or intuition about this?
5. Do you feel punished for being this way when you were a child?

Children with Initial Reaction Difficulties

Practice

Practice is the key word. Parents who have children with difficulties in new situations are best off practicing ahead of time. Annie, the mother of 3-year-old Brenda, who was fearful going to nursery school, was advised by the wise nursery school headmaster to practice getting to the school before the year started. So Annie and Brenda used the exact route a couple of times before nursery began. They dressed as if it were a school day, got into the car, and drove slowly toward the school. Annie pointed out familiar landmarks along the way. These run-throughs eased Brenda's mind tremendously. It was such a success, the exercise helped Annie see how practice could help Brenda's initial reactions in many other situations.

Discuss Solutions Together

As children move beyond the earliest years, they are fully capable of coming up with solutions that will ease the anxiety of situations.

For example, Leora was frightened of her first school bus experience. This was consistent with her usual difficulty in new situations. Instead of getting frustrated with Leora, Mom was encouraged by the school's guidance counselor to have a discussion with her daughter ahead of time. "Ask her," the counselor advised, "what she imagines will be difficult." Leora surprised Mom with questions as to details that many adults don't think of: "Where do I sit? Whom do I sit with? What do I do if there are no seats left?" Once they began talking more concretely about the new situation, many solutions became apparent to Leora and her mother.

The same kind of preparation worked with Gabe, who was apprehensive before going on a play date with a new friend. Gabe did not jump into such situations easily but was able to discuss some of the specific difficulties he imagined might happen. Once voiced with a patient adult, the problems were not so imposing that they couldn't be addressed. He and his dad came up with ways to respond to difficulties—sharing toys or what to do if his new pal became too bossy.

Children Who Have Trouble Adapting

Self-Examination

The most important change a parent can make is to look closely at the number of transitions in a given day. After going through her weekly calendar, Amanda recognized just how many transitions she had been expecting from her son, William. His overbooked calendar looked like a page taken from the appointment book of a top executive of a major corporation. Amanda soon understood that William's difficulty moving from one activity to the other might have less to do with disrespect than it did with his own inborn discomfort about transitioning. She was then much more cooperative as to the schoolteacher's recommendation that she cut down William's extracurricular activities. Within 2 weeks of having only one or two after-school activities, William became a much more pleasant child to be around and Amanda became a much less difficult parent to deal with.

Record Meltdowns

Most children who have problems adapting don't randomly run into trouble. When parents begin to accept a child's hardwiring, they also become more open to the idea that certain scenarios trigger more difficulties. I've asked countless parents and teachers to record meltdowns, and weeks or months later they've come back actually enthusiastic about the patterns they find. It is obvious why they would be enthusiastic—the patterns we recognize almost always lead to fairly simple solutions.

Casey, an 8-year-old who had difficulty during the afternoon in particular, was discovered by her teacher to be most vulnerable right after a hard math lesson. The solution was not to fight Casey's lack of resilience but to go with it. All it took was a moment or two of downtime after math in the classroom to have a happier and more cooperative child for the rest of the school day.

Calendar Check

We take for granted just how frazzled the whole family's schedule can be. But a child who has difficulties adapting is often a barometer of family overscheduling. The following technique, used by many professionals I know, is extremely simple and helpful:

Ask Mom to bring in the family's monthly or weekly calendar, and go over it together. Circle in red the activities that are child centered. This is a truly enlightening exercise for parents—they often realize how much they're asking of themselves and the children. This also helps the helping professional—he or she finds out in a very concrete way just what kind of pressure the family lives with.

Children with High Activity Levels

Structure

Parents must learn the art of "chunking," which means organizing activities into smaller amounts of time or smaller spaces. The more time is left unstructured or the larger and less contained a space is, the greater the activity level of such a child. David, the parent of highly active Alvin, learned from his playgroup teacher to set up smaller play spaces with fewer toys in an area. This was quite different from what he had been doing—allowing Alvin to run free and equipping the playroom with too many toys. Jack and Samantha also discovered that postdinnertime mayhem with their two boys could be greatly reduced. They began to structure activities that would last for brief amounts of time and opted to play in an enclosed area, such as a part of their backyard. Another parent, Claire, realized after our discussion that Ina, her daughter, was much less active after she ran herself ragged in vigorous, exhausting play time.

Vigilance

Help parents become more observant about activities or stimulation that trigger higher activity levels in their kids. There are a number of less obvious stimulants that professionals should be aware of (see the accompanying box).

Ways to Reduce High Activity Levels

Pay attention to:

1. Diet—Food coloring and additives have been implicated in overactivity of children.
2. Allergies—Milk and wheat have been linked to kids' increased activity.
3. TV and video games—Both are associated in some kids with excess activity and restlessness.
4. Play date combinations—Certain pairings invariably increase aimless activity of children.
5. Constructive criticism—Too much gets under many kids' skins, causing restlessness and higher levels of angry activity.

Children Who Are Tenacious

The research with tenacious children shows that it is highly ineffective to engage in head-to-head power struggles with such a child. The idea is, as often as possible, not to get caught in linear escalations. The following is an example of such a linear escalation:

PARENT: I want to turn the TV off now.

CHILD: No.

PARENT: You must turn it off now.

CHILD: (*Ignores parent.*)

PARENT: I'm going to turn it off for you!

CHILD: (*Screams. Runs into the parents' room, turns on parents' TV, and then locks the door.*)

It is easy to see how these interactions can infuriate a parent who doesn't understand tenacity for what it is—a temperamental characteristic. Chronic power struggles are typical with such kids, so use the following guidelines:

Pick and Choose Battles

The most important technique is the one I mentioned in Chapter 1: Help a parent become more aware of the repetitive dances that go on around the house. As I describe in that chapter, ask a parent to keep a brief log of conflictual interactions. The idea is to get Mom or Dad to really think before acting, to cut down on what family therapists call "reactivity." Diminish head-to-head struggles with tenacious children. Stick mainly to those necessary for physical safety and the demands of scheduling.

For example, Francine regularly got into power struggles with her tenacious daughter, Ryan. When she first approached a counselor, Francine believed that every battle was necessary in order to teach good character. The counselor assured Francine that lack of respect was not Ryan's problem but, rather, that she was overdosing on struggles with her mother—issues that really did not hold such import for the future. The counselor asked Francine to keep a list outlining a day of power struggles between the two. Francine came in the next week rather shocked, for the list included battles over outfits that matched, hair done in just the right way, and impeccable table manners. Of the many confrontations, Francine realized, only Ryan's aggression towards siblings and her backtalk truly mattered. It was astonishing how much the entire family settled down as Francine focused on the issues that made a difference.

Limited Choice

The limited choice technique was made famous by the hypnotist Milton Erikson. When Erikson would put people into trance, he'd say, "Do you want to go into a trance now, or in two minutes." Either way, Erikson got the subject to implicitly agree that he or she was eventually going to enter a trance. The same technique works with children: "What do you want to put on first—your socks or your shirt?" Either way, a child, even a tenacious one, feels that there is some choice. It makes no difference (or it should make no difference to a parent) which the child chooses.

Francine gave Ryan limited choices, either one of which she could live with. For example, Ryan was allowed to choose between two different shirts and two or three pants or skirts and a couple of pants or skirts the night before. These choices gave Ryan a sense of autonomy and Mom the sense of control that she needed to feel comfortable.

Walk Away

Whenever it is physically safe, parents need to take a time out from their tenacious children. Art, the father of an incredibly tenacious, hard-negotiating 7-year-old son, Willy, finally understood the need to disengage. He realized that he was not only going to lose many battles with his tough-as-nails son but that he'd be much better off creating some distance before fights got out of hand. Encouraged by Willy's teacher, who had had much experience with being pushed, Art began to respect his own signals that he'd had enough and learned how to tell Willy when he needed a break. At first (as is typical of kids), Willy followed him into the next room, but Art stuck to his guns, closed the door, and even locked it behind him. This change in Art's attitude and approach did not turn Willy into an easy, compliant child, but it significantly cut down on the number of angry battles between the two. And Art's resentment over the kind of kid he "was stuck with" disappeared.

Talk Later

Tenacious kids are entirely unreasonable when they have a goal in sight. However, as determined as they are during a battle, tenacious kids are often intelligent enough to be extremely reasonable later on—after the storm has passed. Such was the case with Isabel, an articulate 4-year-old, who would let nothing get in the way of whatever she happened to want at the moment. It was only when her mother, Pam, began discussing these interactions hours later that Isabel became slightly more reasonable. With such questions as "What could you do instead of pushing or hitting me?" and "How do you think I feel when you get so angry?" Isabel and her mom began to develop a repertoire of less hostile alternatives to channel Isabel's inborn tenacity.

Children with Strong Sensory Reactions

Accept

Parents need to understand that with such a child one cannot yell, punish, or order them out of their sensitivity. There is no way around this reality, and most parents respond exceptionally well to this direct feedback. For example, Burt, a loud-talking attorney who had refused to take advice from teachers and even clergymen in his life, became surprisingly cooperative once he understood that his son, Eddie, was a sensitive child and simply needed to be treated differently. I said to Burt that Eddie could not be yelled at in the same way that another child might. I further suggested that Burt start practicing how to speak more slowly and quietly to the boy. Yelling was an indulgence, I told Burt, and was absolutely no good with Eddie. Illustrated by a tempogram the two of us quickly drew up, Burt finally "got" that, much like his estranged wife and his own father, Eddie was not going to develop a thicker skin overnight.

Adapt

Sensitive kids need to have their sensibilities honored. The child who has never been able to tolerate loud noises should be, as much as possible, protected from them. One who cannot abide by certain types of food, rough clothing, etc. needs to have these sensitivities respected. Use your own words to challenge a parent, but communicate the following concept: "Are you going to fight about this for the rest of your life, or are you going to accept these sensitivities and raise the child you have?"

Shape New Behaviors

When parents finally "get" the child they have and in fact have always had, they stop fighting and become more capable of strengthening the child's vulnerabilities. For example, highly sensitive Aaron made major changes when his mom, Estelle, could hear the message, "Stop yelling—talk more slowly!" To help, I taught Estelle to take three deep breaths until she felt calmer and could address Aaron in a less aggressive way. Over a period of months, Aaron began to be less of a "crybaby"; not that his basic temperament had changed significantly, but he was able to listen, cry less, and become much more affectionate toward Estelle. You can imagine how this affected her self esteem and satisfaction as a mother.

Another concept for the professional to learn is that sensitivities can be shaped through good old-fashioned desensitization. Kids who have trouble going to loud, intense movies can conquer this by peeking in for brief periods of time and staying longer as they become more comfortable. New foods can be introduced very, very gradually. For sensitive kids, slowing down the pace will not foster power struggles based on the child's fear.

Children Who Have Difficulties with Mood

Stop Self-Blame

As I described above, parents of children whose mood is less exuberant or whose endurance is not as resilient need to blame themselves less. Chronic disappointment about their supposed incompetence almost guarantees unhappiness at home. For example, Rachael, continuously worried that she had seriously damaged her daughter, Laura, by having gone to work the first few years of the girl's life. Rachael became much less self-critical and more open to suggestions when, after tracing a family history and doing a tempogram, she recognized that Laura's level of exuberance had been different all along from that of her other daughter, Nikki.

More Warmth

The lack of defensiveness on Rachael's part, once this burden of guilt lifted, was remarkable. Less resilient children need more downtime and parental affection. So, Rachael immediately began spending a little extra time with Laura, just doing nothing: hanging out, arts and crafts projects, and other undemanding kinds of activities. These calmed Laura and strengthened the bond between her and Mom. Over a period of a few months, Laura's mood had significantly lifted. She was still not a wildly exuberant child, but she no longer seemed as petulant or sullen.

Teach Optimism

Children who are less resilient can, in fact, be slowly helped to create greater optimism. Researchers such as Martin E. P. Seligman (*The Optimistic Child*, Houghton Mifflin, 1995) have shown that children predisposed to depressive moods often are more vulnerable because of the way they negatively evaluate their own experiences. For example, Gene is a child who could become quite sullen. One summer, an experienced camp counselor majoring in graduate school psychology realized that Gene's self-evaluations were almost always negative. The counselor made an enormous difference in

Gene's life by sitting down with him and intuitively understanding that the boy needed to be more *realistic* about his self-appraisals. "Yes," he would say, "you are not the best at basketball." Gene reacted positively, just as Seligman's research shows, to this realistic feedback. Children with less buoyant moods feel better with realistic feedback than unwarranted compliments such as "You're the best!" or "You're the greatest anyway!" The truth, delivered in a kind way, almost always makes kids feel better. Why? Because it leads to concrete solutions that can help many situations improve: "So, you know," the counselor continued, "I'll take you out for a few minutes every day and practice with you." This approach—realistic feedback, a concrete solution, and action to address the situation—is enormously powerful with children who do not have extra doses of optimism.

*   *   *

Once we can identify the inborn temperament of difficult children, we can help parents with specific recommendations that ease difficulties. Tenacious kids move from being tyrannical to being determined; oversensitive children become more sure of themselves; less adaptable youngsters have fewer meltdowns; and moody kids show greater resilience. These children remain a challenge, but they are no longer simply impossible.

chapter four

Up Against the Wall

Getting Through to Difficult Parents

As professionals we've all met them, whether we are teachers, counselors, community leaders, camp directors, nurses, therapists, or pediatricians: parents who come to us for help with their children but end up viewing us as threats instead of allies. Unpredictably, they greet our advice and the changes we ask of them with resistance and distrust. Maybe they have very strong belief systems that dictate the way things should be done in their families; maybe they are just uninterested or, for unknown reasons, become disengaged from a process that depends on willing collaborators. There's the father who challenges everything suggested by any professional. There's the mother who, with every word or subtle glance, exudes the belief that she and only she will ever know what's best for her child. Or perhaps you've counseled couples who fight so effectively you end up feeling absolutely impotent and beside the point.

Whatever their stripes, they seem to make it impossible for us helping professionals to create any change. Try as we might, we can't seem to get through to them. They are simply "difficult" parents.

Of course, it's not that simple, and rarely is it that hopeless. Over the years, I've discovered several essential factors that are key to getting through to even the most resistant parents. The core issue that makes or breaks us getting through to difficult parents is whether we are able to *empathize* more accurately with them. This chapter addresses the specific problem of how to increase your level of empathy toward parents across all professional situations. I outline how difficult parents can be better understood and what concrete strategies are most effective.

Toward Greater Understanding: Why Culture Makes Parents Difficult

In almost very case, I encounter parents who are unable or unwilling to work with the kind of changes I am asking of them because they feel deeply misunderstood. The major reason parents ask us for help but then reject our efforts is that today's parents are likely to feel unsupported and misunderstood by all sides, including us.

Lack of Support

Society as a whole puts mothers and fathers on the defensive. The last 30 years or so have seen a general erosion of the usual supports that strengthen a parent's authority. Neighborhoods which once provided kinship and friendship systems have broken down. Traditional neighborhoods or small towns replete with ritual structure and tradition extending back for several generations have been replaced by urban sprawl and anonymous big city living. A majority of Americans now live either in cities or in suburban areas.

Despite these demographic changes, community life has made a slight resurgence since the early 1990s. This is shown by increased numbers of church, synagogue, and community organizations, increased membership in community groups such as the Boy Scouts and Girl Scouts, and increased general philanthropic activities. While, indeed, the resurgence of community structures is a welcome change, these new organizations do not make up for the continuing sense of ennui and frenetic disconnection experienced throughout urban and suburban postmodern America. Simply put, these emerging neighborhood structures do not have the authoritative weight that kinship systems and traditional religious organizations once had. This is because most Americans are willing to trade less authority for more freedom. To paraphrase pollster and social commentator George Gallup, Jr.: We want our religious and community life. We just don't want anyone telling us how to live (*Public Perspective*, October/November 1995). His findings were corroborated by research I did interviewing the adults in children's lives: teachers, group leaders, camp owners, day care and nursery directors, and so on. The structural authority that used to exist no longer confers immediate respect on parents, nor does it give them support. For most parents, authority is not a given, it is something that grownups have to earn.

It is extremely important to recognize this lack of everyday support because it increases one's empathy toward mothers and fathers. This can be an antidote against adopting an overly sympathetic attitude toward kids, which only makes parents more defensive and difficult to deal with.

It's All Their Fault

Throughout society, experience tells parents that they are the creators of terrible dysfunction. From the schools to pop culture to the mental health establishment, all fingers of blame point to Mom and Dad—especially Mom. Whether it's for a child being dressed improperly, running inconsiderately up and down the aisles during a concert or having deep psychological problems—the finger of blame is never far from today's parents.

We professionals make our own contribution to difficult parents feeling blamed. Even family therapists don't believe that kids create problems or that they have a significant impact on family life. We have historically suggested that problems between parents are usually the main issue. The child is the symptom-bearer for these dysfunctional forces. In fact, we are proud when we can get kids out of the room to start working with parents on the "real" underlying difficulties. No wonder parents feel we don't understand what they're up against.

We Don't Like Kids

Mothers and fathers often express resentment toward their own kids. Surveys show that between 50% and 70% of adults don't like kids all that much ("We Don't Like Our Kids," *The New York Observer*, July 21, 1997). "They're selfish and rude," say a majority of Americans. Parents may resent children because of how demanding they are and how much they cost—emotionally and economically. There is plenty of evidence to show that the financial expenses of child rearing drain the possibility for a comfortable retirement. With kids not taught to show gratitude—a child-centered culture and kiddie values that urge kids to "Do it," "Take care of Number 1," and expect instant gratification—it's no wonder parents come in unsympathetic to their own children or to our efforts.

As professionals, of course, we can't separate ourselves from the culture we live in. So, whether we were repeatedly taught that mothers and fathers are always to blame for children's problems, whether we inadvertently soak up all the parent-blaming images in the media, or whether we ourselves had difficulties with our own parents, it's hard not to be biased. When mothers and fathers approach us they are likely to be faced with the same impatience and stereotyping that exists everywhere else. We *are*, as parents, correctly suspect, willing to blame them for their kids' problems.

Where does this leave you—the eager professional who wants to help? How can teachers enlist greater cooperation from parents; how can guidance and pastoral counselors be more accessible and effectively authoritative with parents; how can group leaders and community organizers be more effective and inspiring in their leadership? The answer requires reservoirs of empathy and a bag of tricks to help "difficult" parents. How to instill in parents the sense that they are being understood sufficiently to create a *readiness for change* is the subject of this chapter.

Creating Readiness for Change

Find Out What Mom or Dad Wants

Several decades ago, Barbara Lerner, a researcher studying psychotherapy clinics, discovered a very simple truth: clients dropped out of counseling for one basic reason—the professional didn't listen to what they wanted. My experience as director of a not-for-profit clinic validates the truth of Lerner's finding. Unless we find out what a parent wants to change, in all likelihood we will never see him or her again.

The most powerful way to bridge the gap is also the most obvious. You need to ask. You literally must say to mothers and fathers, "What can I do to help you? What would make *you* feel better?" This is quite different than a righteous, moral position—that we know, that we're there to tell others the *absolute right thing to do.* We should offer advice, but not without making sure we're responding to a parent's need. We must be clear that we are interested in helping mothers or fathers get what they want. When you state this out loud, "Mom, Dad, I am here to help *you,*" the built-in resistance many parents feel diminishes. It starts to be replaced by growing awareness that he or she has found an ally in you.

Here are some concrete needs parents might have and how you might acknowledge your willingness to collaborate in reaching these goals.

• *"I want you to fix my child."* This has always been seen as a surefire indicator of a parent's resistance. But now I think just the opposite: Mom and Dad are usually onto something. They are frustrated or angry, but they also recognize a real problem in their child. When you hear such a request, *don't dismiss it.* Instead refocus, as in "Tell me exactly what you mean." For example, the mother and father of an 8-year-old came to see me. Regardless of how well their child seemed to be doing in school, he still acted up a lot at home. "The teachers say we're crazy," Mom complained, "but we believe that something is wrong with our child. He has tantrums too quickly when plans don't go the way he expects them to—Please help us fix him."

You need to hear the specific ways a parent wants you to fix a child: some goals are more reasonable than others, but all must be heard and acknowledged.

• *"I want to feel appreciated by my kids."* Increasingly, I hear this from both mothers and fathers. Lack of appreciation is one reason many parents have underlying feelings of resentment toward children. Daily, I hear stories of parents who go out of their way doing child-centered activities without feeling sufficient gratitude coming from the kids. One such incident occurred with some children during a visit to a very crowded and shockingly expensive amusement park. After hours of catering to the kids' needs and going on one frightening ride after the other, one of the kids had a complete melt down when her parents would not get her a tee-shirt at the park's gift shop. "How could our daughter not focus on what we *had* done," her parents wondered, "rather than focus on the tiny detail that we were not willing to give to her." Lack of appreciation fuels a huge amount of chronic resentment and anger in child-centered parents.

This is not unusual and is a great source of resentment in parents of modern kids. It's important to show that you recognize this gratitude deprivation from the parents' perspective; and it is especially critical that you openly appreciate what an effort has been made on a child's behalf. Appreciation is exactly what has been missing for most parents, and your acknowledgment of *whatever* feels good or noble or earnest is an important step toward creating collaboration. Teachers can well understand gratitude deprivation. So many have told me that they feel an ongoing lack of appreciation from both parents and kids. As one teacher put it at an in-house seminar I was giving, "Parents never seem to realize that this is more than just a 9–5 job for us and that occasionally we, too, need to be thanked. The money alone can't make up for how hard it is, and it never will."

• *"Help me to see that I'm not crazy."* This usually means: "Help me see that the way I'm handling things is not totally wrong and that I'm not a complete failure." As Allison told me, "Other parents seem to be able to handle several children. I have this one girl who manages to push all my buttons and drives me absolutely nuts. She's so intense, and she has an answer for everything. She never lets go until she wins. I become totally unhinged by her." In these situations, the counselor should find genuine ways that the parents have not been entirely wrong headed but instead have been more reasonable than not.

For example, I reminded Allison that while I believed her frustration was merited, she'd still been able to help her daughter have friends and do well in school. Now we would work on ways to be less reactive at home.

- *"I want to get closer to my child."* The entire mental health profession developed out of a parent-blaming model. For decades, theory taught thousands upon thousands of therapists, counselors, and even clergy the pathological effects of overly close parent–(especially mother–child bonds. The pathologization of connection is obvious when it comes to counselors and therapists, but teachers too are wary of what can be viewed as overly enmeshed parent–child dyads. Whether it manifests itself in their stance toward parents involved in homework, rigid boundaries between the classroom and home, or a paucity of information that teachers share with mothers and fathers, it is painfully apparent that teachers also are prone to negatively label connection as enmeshment, bonds as overprotection. Given what I've just described, it is no surprise that wanting to get closer to one's child may be labeled as overly intrusive or enmeshed. This value judgment may have been true decades ago when family members were so close—in physical and emotional proximity—that they were virtually under each other's skin. But now, with life moving so fast, kids and parents live in parallel and sometimes distant universes. Many parents who are in trouble with their kids really *do* want to feel closer to them. They want kids to express more affection. They want kids to tell them more. The truth is that at some point earlier on most parents and kids were in love with each other. Sadly, along the way, they fell out of love and became adversaries. Parents and kids (even teens) want to recapture some of that feeling. This is a legitimate need in our fragmented times.

For example, Susan complained about her 11-year-old daughter, Patricia: "She keeps to herself or only wants to talk to her friends. She gives me one-word answers, and it seems we can go weeks without exchanging much in the way of conversation except about the logistics of life." Susan's unhappiness with this situation is not unusual. Modern family life being what it is, we often feel like strangers to our own children, like ships passing in the night. This is a feeling that needs validation, not the judgments of a society all too quick to label and negatively interpret such need.

State Your Intentions

The second step in creating readiness for change is to clearly state your intention that you want to help. This is a simple but revolutionary change in our tradition. Most of us were taught that people ought to come up with answers themselves. More insidiously, the idea of saying—or even feeling—that you would like to help has been traditionally frowned upon. An old supervisor of mine would publicly denigrate such obvious desires to do good with the worst possible label (in his mind): we were trying to be caseworkers! So, it is far from surprising that we don't always state our professional and personal intention to be of service—what an important factor to leave out of the human equation.

State that your goal is, within reason, to try to help parents get what they want. I say within reason because, whatever your role—teacher, guidance counselor, group leader, and so on—you need to expand your ability to empathize and collaborate with the parents you meet. Here are some ways:

1. "I'm going to try to give you what you need."
2. "I'm going to try to help you feel less crazy."
3. "I'm going to try to help your child love and respect you more."
4. "I'm going to try to help you feel more competent."

We Will Do It Together

You need to state that you will work *together* with parents. This immediately clears the often-adversarial atmosphere. When mothers and fathers hear you say, "We're going to try to collaborate," most parents will sense a new approach. They will say to themselves:

1. "You're not ordering me around—telling me what to do."
2. "You're not blaming me."
3. "You don't think I'm totally at fault."
4. "You think we can work on this together."

It's a generous offer, and it's exactly what mothers and fathers need to hear. Remember: with no extended family, fewer institutional supports, a schism between home and school, they've been hearing just the opposite.

I will never forget the woman who, after listening to the support that she could expect to get from me said, "For the first time, I don't feel so alone; it's almost like I had my old neighborhood back."

Challenging Parents

As a field, we have tried to seduce parents. We adopt a relaxing style ingenuously, congratulate them on their successes, and positively reframe behaviors they've previously thought unacceptable. Somehow, though, "difficult" parents sense the inauthenticity of our technique, and this phony professional demeanor often doesn't seem to be enough. In order to get through, after empathy and a spirit of collaboration have been offered, a direct challenge must follow. Helping kids is, after all, dependent on getting parents to try new behaviors. Here's how:

1. Be clear that you're after change. After bridging the rift between professional and parent, helping a mother or father believe that we are on their side, a *challenge* must always follow. By challenge I mean saying, in one way or another: " To make things better, *you're* going to have to change." There is no way around this direct challenge, nor should there be. Find the words and phrases that are suitable to the particular parent you're facing, and then be clear about your goal—you are going to attempt to make things better by encouraging at least some change on mother's or father's (or both parents') part.

2. Know what you stand for. Challenging parents means knowing what you stand for. This is not easy. Even teachers and guidance counselors who have not had the notion of professional neutrality drummed into their heads have been repeatedly reminded to be ever watchful of overemphasizing their own values to the parents and kids they work with. Administrators in schools and social agencies also discourage their teachers and clinicians from being overly opinionated, for fear of parental reactions in this litigious society. After years of professional neutrality on all fronts, then, it is not that simple to stand for certain principles that we know will help kids do well in life. In Chapter 11, I describe in greater detail the child-rearing tenets proven to be essential for healthy development. The idea of challenge is that instead of maintaining a stance of neutrality, we are not afraid to make what's important explicit to a parent. This "I–thou" exchange, as Martin Buber called it, is central to helping parents feel supported by another human being, a real presence in the room.

For example, parents may approach you to help create better communication between them and their child. After gathering information through some of the techniques described in Chapter 1, you'll need to make an evaluation about what you believe is appropriate to change. Maybe the parents' complaint is really not warranted. Perhaps it's adequate communication for the child's age or communicative style. But, more likely, parents have a realistic sense that the child *is* too quiet— they just don't know how to make it better. Rather than being obtuse or patronizing, it must be said directly: "I will help you find out more about your child, *but it will require that you learn how to listen better.*" Or, in another situation, a father might complain that his child is not respectful enough. For example, Abe complained that Sandy, his daughter, answered back in a way he thought inappropriate for any child, especially his. Unfortunately, Abe's way of dealing with this was to raise his voice in such a harsh, out-of-control manner that Sandy immediately began screaming and crying herself, often calling Abe even worse names. While one could certainly empathize with Abe's desire for more respect, he was not going to get it from this child by being harsh and frightening. The challenge would be, "Abe, you want your child to respect you more and be less rude. But this may mean that you will need to yell less and lose it less often."

Creating Change: Five Principles

Many of us child professionals ask people to take steps that are much too big. We push them to be different from who they are; we forget the belief systems and values that predate us and extend way into the past. We do all this mainly because we have the view that clients exist only in the moments we actually see them. During my training, this narcissistic perspective always amazed me. Some of my supervisors would watch a 30-second videotaped segment of a family therapy session and draw sweeping conclusions about the parents' entire character based on this tiny slice of life. Because of this tradition, it may be hard to imagine what people are like and what they must face when we're not around. Especially with diffi- cult parents, the complexity of their lives often eludes us: they may well have more loving aspects than we can possibly imagine, or more extraordinary adversity than they can possibly handle.

Creating change means that we see mothers and fathers clearly enough so that we don't ask too much or too little of them. This empathy is necessary to transform a difficult parent into one whose mind is open enough that new behavior is possible. The following are five key principles you must remember:

1. Changes Must Be Consistent with Who the Parents Are

It is central in fostering change that it be consistent with who a par- ent is. A mother, Susan, whom I met after a terrible family tragedy taught me this. She told me in no uncertain terms that regardless of what I thought was better for her 13-year-old daughter, "I cannot behave in a way that is inconsistent with who I am." Specifically, Susan deeply felt that self-expression (vaunted by most mental health professionals as a sign of health) would never be more im- portant than being a kind person. Susan was warning me that she could not abide a daughter who would be emotionally open but not respectful of other people's feelings. Perhaps because of the tragic circumstances surrounding the family (or being a parent myself), I knew Susan was onto something.

Rather than the *principle of consistency* being a hindrance, I have found just the opposite. Since I've learned to be more respectful of who a parent is, mothers and fathers have been more willing to listen to me about what they need to change. For example, Al and Tina, parents of a young adolescent, Johnny, discovered that he had been smoking pot. They called me up in a frenzy. Al and Tina wanted to know: should they confront Johnny; should they pretend nothing happened and put it on the back burner for a couple of days; should they create an immediate consequence? Al and Tina are very "up-front" people. I knew them well and realized that they could not hold themselves back. So, in keeping with the principle of consistency, I said, "You can't *not* bring it up! That's not you. If you try to be phony, it will end up backfiring. Just try not to explode when you do bring it up." With this synthesis of validation and challenge, Al and Tina did, in fact, talk to Johnny that night when they were a lot calmer.

2. All Change Begins as "False-Self" Change

The moment of trying new strategies is one of mixed emotions—usually hope is intertwined with skepticism and a sense that the new behavior is "phony." It feels, to use an old psychoanalytic expression, like a "false-self" experience. For example, the parent who reflexively yells, one who always lectures, or another who comforts a sobbing child will find it extremely strange to suddenly lower his or her voice, refrain from lecturing, or leave a distraught child alone. This sense of weirdness comes from going against natural tendencies and entering unfamiliar territory. When the desired response follows—a child listens or calms himself down—the parent gets to experience firsthand *why* a strategy is helpful. At that point, he or she becomes truly motivated to try the strategy again. The second time it no longer feels as false. Help a parent be ready for the strangeness of change by explaining the false-self phenomenon.

3. Aim for Change That Will Cause "Just-Tolerable Anxiety" for the Parent

The mistake we make challenging parents is that we invariably ask for too much. "Too much" translates into a variety of reasons: anxiety about the unknown, resentment because the parent feels justifiably provoked by the child, a sense of discouragement from numerous failures, or child-rearing belief systems that span generations. Aiming for change that will cause just-tolerable anxiety is both challenging and respectful of who a parent is.

For example, Thelma, a mother, I recently met, was in the habit of saying to her son, "You're such a bad eater, you're killing me." As the helping professional, I would, of course, like Thelma to stop uttering these dire warnings. But Thelma says, "Hey, this is pretty good, because at least I'm not holding a knife to him like my mother—may she rest in peace—did with me when *I* refused to eat."

In this case, as in any other just-tolerable anxiety means challenging the parents in a way that increases the likelihood of a success scenario. Here's how:

a. Establish a baseline. Find out how many times a day, a week, or a month the target behavior occurs. In Thelma's case, she made these alarming statements three or four times a week. In another situation, in which a parent might nag, put down, or "lose it" with a child, you might find an entirely different baseline.

b. Establish an alternative behavior. Thelma and I explored what she could say that would relieve her frustration and also create an impact. At first, Thelma had a hard time coming up with any other response. But after a while she settled on saying, "I need you to eat. It's extremely upsetting to me if you don't." Often, several meetings may be focused simply on finding alternative solutions. For example, Clara complained that her 5-year-old daughter, Debra, got easily bored. Debra would reject all of Clara's suggestions and stick with activities for only brief periods of time before wanting to zone out in front of the TV. This disturbed Clara enormously, but she'd run out of ideas. So, it took several sessions to come up with a number of other solutions for the boredom problem. Clara finally settled on creating with Debra a chart of possible activities for Debra when there was nothing else to do, and Debra could choose from this master list herself.

c. Be specific about how often to try a new behavior. It is not enough to say, "Ok, give it a try." Parents need specificity—child rearing is such a messy business. Thelma decided that she could give up her extreme warnings three times a week. I did not agree. Why? Because a good rule of thumb in creating just-tolerable anxiety is to go with *less* rather than more. When Thelma immediately offered to give up making those alarming statements several times, my response was to emphasize how difficult this would be. We eventually settled on just once a week.

Another example: I had to be very specific with Phoebe about her college freshman son Allan's sporadic phone calls from school. It was not enough to say to Phoebe, "When you feel that sufficient time has passed, give Allan a call." For several reasons, such a vague directive would have led to confusion. We needed to be much more specific: if a call was made too early in the morning, her son wouldn't want to talk; if she asked too many detailed questions, Allan would feel she was being an overcontrolling mother; if she called too late, he would probably be out and Phoebe would worry more. After much back-and-forth discussion, the specific solution was that Phoebe would call every week or so during the early evening hours. Allan was most communicative then, and more responsive to Mom's calling to just say hello. This specificity made all the difference between success and failure.

d. Explore what might get in the way of change. "What," I asked Thelma, "do you think will make it tough to stop getting so emotional?" People know themselves a lot better than we do. This makes it important that we ask them to imagine the details of daily life that will make any change hard. At first Thelma responded, "Nothing! I know I can do this." I again opted for the least rather than the most anxiety and said, "I'm not sure; can you imagine anything that would get in the way?" Thelma experienced my caution as a validation of how difficult change really would be and, after a thoughtful moment, admitted, "You know, if my son has had an active day, then refuses to eat hardly any supper, I know it will be hard for me not to get upset."

Getting back to Phoebe, I asked her, "What might make it tough to stay away from bugging Allan about the details of his life?" This was an important question. Phoebe immediately recognized she would get triggered if Allan was vague or refused to say much, or if he wouldn't nail down a time to talk on the phone again. An ounce of prevention here was worth a pound of cure. Sure enough, Allan responded in his typically superficial way during the next conversation. Only this time Phoebe was not so easily provoked.

It is essential for you to take this more cautious route. Even less flexible parents like Thelma feel validated and a little more open to change.

e. Reach an agreement, or don't ask for change. Many years ago in my initial family therapy training, we used to shake hands with a parent and a child after they agreed to try out new behavior. One doesn't have to literally shake hands, but making an "agreement ritual," either verbally, by writing it down, or by sealing it with a handshake says to a parent that you're taking this all very seriously. Thelma and I verbally agreed that *once* in the coming week, when she felt herself about to lose it, instead of using any life-or-death phrases, she would simply say, "This is getting me very upset."

Another illustration: Clara agreed that one time during the next week she would let Debra just "hang out"—watch TV or lay around the family room. It was important for us to make this verbal agreement together, for otherwise, given the intense pace of their lives, it would be forgotten or ignored.

Another example involved Mr. Parsons at a school in an urban center. I was called in to consult with him because he had been repeatedly arguing with kids in front of their classmates. My work with him was not unlike with the parents I see: we needed to agree on a small but doable change. In Mr. Parsons's case, we reached an understanding that he would attempt to not yell once or twice a day when he felt the urge, but rather would ask the child to leave the classroom and discuss it later. After thinking about it, Mr. Parsons admitted that because this class was so aggravating to him, the most realistic agreement he could make was to try this one time a day. To me this was more than acceptable because it was realistic and reaching an agreement in this way ensured that he would give "time outs" a chance. In fact, as I found out weeks later, after a couple of highly successful attempts at holding his yelling back, Mr. Parsons got enough positive reinforcement to spontaneously cut down yelling at a much quicker pace.

4. Help Parents Understand That the Assigned Tasks Are Probably Going to Fail

Most tasks and homework assignments are doomed to failure. Not only is this expected, but it actually helps us know what other hidden and perhaps more important issues need to be addressed with the parent. No matter how carefully you follow the above suggestions, more than likely some tasks are going to fail for the following reasons:

   a. **Harried lives.** The most likely cause for failed homework assignments is that we don't understand how overscheduled, overworked, and frazzled people's lives really are. In one family, we had agreed on Mom or Dad spending 15 extra minutes per night with each of the two children. Little did I realize how unrealistic this idea was. Given the family's overscheduling, it was impossible for them to find a half hour of extra time each night. Several weeks later, a little wiser, we agreed on 15 minutes extra with each child *once a week*. It may not seem like much, but this was the just-tolerable level of anxiety that these parents could manage and it began the process of change.

   b. **Family-of-origin obstacles.** A failed task often expresses an unresolved issue dating back to the parent's own family of origin. For example, as Thelma pointed out, she had been involved in a power struggle over food with her own mother. Al and Tina, who discovered their son smoking pot, had both been raised by parents who never talked openly with them. It was understandable, in light of their backgrounds, that asking them to say nothing would have been like demanding that they repeat a negative history.

In another family, the idea that the kids ought to be allowed *some* TV or video time, which seemed to me entirely reasonable and at least worth a try, to these particular parents sounded almost primitive. Though Mom and Dad intellectually understood that their kids needed to be part of the pop culture, they had both been raised in highly academic, striving families. The idea that they were now going to allow their children to watch a couple of sitcoms and teenage soap operas a week may have seemed momentarily reasonable in my presence but, given their family history, turned out to be an almost ridiculous suggestion.

c. Personal demons. Failed tasks often founder on the hidden rocks of parents' individual problems. Sometimes the most minor suggestion about a parent changing his or her behavior with a child can reveal extraordinary circumstances. For example, Linda, a mother of several grade-schoolers, came to me complaining about her sloppy children. No amount of nagging, reminding, or punishing seemed to get them to pick up after themselves. As I tried to create a task aimed at cutting down on some of her criticism around the house, Linda threw up her hands and finally admitted, "I think its harder for me to stay on top of myself—after I've had that third glass of wine." What had started out as a simple homework assignment had ended up leading to Linda's long-standing problem with alcohol.

In another family, Joe, a father of two adolescent girls, complained about how distant both daughters had become since entering adolescence. As I gathered information, it became clear that his loud and abrasive responses to them had something to do with their distance. When, after a few tries, Joe couldn't soften his aggressive tone, his wife told me, and Joe admitted, that he'd hated his own father's wishy-washy tone during his childhood. He'd rather be a tough, feared dad than a Milquetoast-like dismissed one.

A final, very dramatic example: Yvonne complained that her two children made her irritable. Each week Yvonne came back having "failed" at adopting a more relaxed view toward their fairly minor and run-of-the-mill transgressions. In passing one day, Yvonne asked me whether it was OK to smoke during our meetings. I said she couldn't because I was allergic to cigarettes. She replied, "Well, I think I ought to tell you that I have a bit of a smoking habit." "How much," I asked, never for a moment imagining what I would hear. "Five and a half packs a day," Yvonne said almost off-handedly, "and I drink a little coffee, too." "Yeah, how much?" I asked again, this time slightly more prepared for her response. "About twenty-five cups a day," Yvonne admitted somewhat sheepishly.

I cannot tell you how typical my experience with Yvonne has turned out to be over the years. So many times I've asked parents to do things that they have been unable to manage. I then find out months later, even years later, that there is a hidden individual issue often involving a serious life experience or condition that hasn't been addressed. The major ones are the following: controlled substance abuse, violence or sexual abuse in a parent's history, untreated affective disorders, moderate obsessive–compulsive syndromes, and panic attacks. I now look for these red flag indicators of a more serious issue:

Although we have found a reasonable agreed-upon task—

- It triggers a just-tolerable level of anxiety.
- The parents cannot, for whatever reasons, give it a try.
- We spend several weeks modifying the task to better fit the parents' specific situation.
- The parents keep engaging in behavior they *know* is ineffective.

In such cases, I meet with each parent individually or, if appropriate, ask in front of his or her spouse, "Is there anything going on that I don't know about yet?" Invariably, I hear about hidden issues that are keeping the parent "difficult" and unable to change.

Following Up

A major question counselors have is whether to bring up a task at the next meeting or follow the parent's lead. These steps will help you take charge without being overly directive:

1. Ask how the week went. Especially in households where there is a lot of tension, it is important to get a general sense of the mood since the last time you met. You want to make sure that there have been no major fights or troubling events. For example, Arden and Bill had come to see me for help with their child's difficulty handing in homework. Unfortunately, the mood of the house was so dependent on whether the couple had had a fight that any homework assignment was dependent on how things had gone between them. Checking in with all families about the general tone of the household is an essential first question.

2. Ask if anything new has come up. Sometimes people are so compliant, or such "good" soldiers, that they bring up the homework assignment despite extraordinary events. Once such person, Maureen, immediately whipped out her notes about a task that we'd agreed upon. After listening to her describe the events in a muted manner, I asked, "Are you sure nothing else of importance has occurred?" It turned out that Maureen's husband, Marvin, had been fired—a detail she did not think to bring up because, in her mind, homework from the "authority" took precedence.

3. Now it's time to ask about the homework. After checking in about the past week and addressing mood changes you sense, refer to your notes and ask in a nonjudgmental way, "So how did it go?" The communication should send the message that you didn't expect it to go perfectly or smoothly. Remember, what's important is not success or failure; what counts is where the parent may have run into trouble or how you may have misjudged the homework's difficulty.

4. Reassessing the just-tolerable level of anxiety. The process of change is furthered enormously when parents begin to understand that failure does not mean the situation is hopeless or that you will give up. What it *does* mean, however, is that the task needs to be readjusted. The just-tolerable level of anxiety has not been found.

John and Myra came back after a homework assignment dejected over the fact that they could not find 10 minutes a night to discuss what had happened with the kids. My accepting tone helped them understand that perhaps we had overreached in our expectations. In fact, finding a couple of minutes two or three times a week was more consistent with their lives and ability to deal with intimacy. This was not a failure on their part; it was an avoidable mistake on mine—a detour necessary to begin a more authentic process of change.

*   *   *

Following these suggestions about creating a readiness for change and challenges can encourage the most difficult parents to become sympathetic, even heroic, figures. This not only leads to greater change, it also makes the work we do and the relationships we create feel far more collaborative than adversarial.

chapter five Gut Responses

Handling Anger, Outrage, Sexuality, and Other "Unprofessional" Feelings

The work we professionals do with families and their children can be incredibly provocative. Parents regularly trigger the least attractive sides of our personalities. Counselors, teachers, therapists, doctors, clergy, caseworkers—the list is endless—have come to me aghast at the kinds of intense reactions they've experienced toward the very people they were expected to help. Indeed, if most of us were entirely honest, we would be forced to admit that not a day, sometimes not a meeting, goes by without experiencing one or another feeling that seems, at best, to be highly unprofessional. This lack of emotional discipline on our part can extend into our behavior as well.

For example, several years ago, I made a common yet amateurish error with a young couple I was seeing for the first time. I interpreted their problem before we had established any kind of working relationship and way before they were ready to hear my opinion. The couple did not return and, feeling terrible about making this mistake, I decided to call and apologize. While on the phone, I told them that, because the session had been essentially useless, I wouldn't charge them for the time. Feeling a need to reassure them about this, I found myself loudly ripping up their check, providing a sound effect on the other side of the phone. This extra effort to concretely take responsibility seemed more than a little bizarre to me. Why had I done it? After all, I hadn't been that terrible. I'd just made an honest mistake.

A month later, I spoke to the couple's new therapist and was startled to learn that the major issue of treatment was their need to have *their* parents take responsibility for child-rearing errors. In particular, the couple wanted their parents to show contrition by loaning— with no strings attached—start-up money for a new house. I then saw that, through a sweeping series of "errors," I had unwittingly expressed the dynamics of this couple's underlying problem. In short, I had reenacted the problem itself.

To avoid being swallowed up whole by a family's turbulent emotions or a child's intense style—what individual therapists call "countertransference"—many professionals who work with parents and kids institute various safeguards including one-way mirrors, supervisors, a working team, teacher and counselor support groups, and so on. While various techniques may help us stay clearheaded enough to do a good job, their use rests on two assumptions: the first is that we have the luxury of working with a team or one-way mirror when, in this productivity-conscious era, most of us are likely to be alone—fragile and vulnerable facing intense family emotions; the second is that experiencing these emotions is bad and should be avoided at all costs. I would like to suggest instead that many emotionally based counseling and teaching "errors" we make can be vital guides in our work, often pointing with uncanny precision to central issues we've missed that will actually help work with parents and kids.

Why Errors Are Inevitable

In 1972, psychoanalyst Edgar A. Levenson wrote *The Fallacy of Understanding* (Basic Books; reprinted by Aronson, 1995). In this book, and many subsequent articles that have had a profound impact on the world of psychoanalysis, Levenson describes how therapists cannot help repeating aspects of a patient's unresolved family relationships. So, for example, despite our best intentions with a client whose mother has been neglectful or harsh, we find ourselves at times acting inexplicably inattentive, indifferent, or unempathic. The unconscious pull exerted by a patient to "transform" (Levenson's word) his or her therapist into acting out underlying family dynamics is so compelling that no amount of precautionary safeguards can entirely prevent it.

Levenson does not regard this transformation of the therapist as an evil to be sidestepped whenever possible but, rather, as an unsurpassed therapeutic tool. Recognizing how we've been transformed can cast a here-and-now spotlight on the often elusive beliefs and interactive processes that sustain a parent's worldview and his or her approach to a problem. Pulling ourselves out of these transformations can be the crucial moments in our work, offering new points of departure for mothers and fathers.

For example, Helen, a supervisee in my counseling program, during the first session with a set of overwhelmed parents and their two unruly children, gave the family *six* homework assignments, *all due the following week*. She also reported feeling somewhat frazzled in the meeting and being unable to pay any attention to what the children were saying. Helen had always been a cool, clear thinker, an excellent listener, and philosophically opposed to being overly directive with families. Believing that this uncharacteristic response might be useful, I asked her to mention, during the next meeting, that she had been too demanding with the assignments and to find out if anyone else in the family also made unrealistic and compulsive demands.

As it turned out, both mother and father were driven, highly compulsive people themselves. Mother constantly created lists of tasks for father and the children, and father, while ignoring her lists, made the lives of his work subordinates miserable with his equally lengthy and elaborate requirements. Both spent so much time directing that they had long since lost effective control over their children, who, feeling overwhelmed and ignored, were always on the verge of rebellion.

Helen's unwitting transformation into a taskmaster was a critical sign showing her the way to engage these parents. Transformations usually reflect aspects of relationships taken for granted by family members that are often the most personal parts of family life. When Helen briefly enacted the problem and they recognized it, she not only created an intense connection with Mom and Dad, she brought into focus what had been mysteriously ailing them. Counseling could then evolve from "fixing" everyone (a continuation of the problem) to discussing how miserable it was to live in a high-pressure environment so pervasive it had always been invisible to them.

This application of Levenson's idea of transformation to interventions with mothers, fathers, and children is highly instructive. First, these transformations happen immediately—sometimes within the first phone contact. For example, within the first few minutes talking, I found myself acting extremely hassled and curt toward a mother. Later, I found out mom's chief complaint was how rude and frenzied her daughter acted toward *her*! Thus, subtle transformations often occur within moments of meeting people. Second, the *way* we're transformed is a vital diagnostic indicator that helps us sift through the enormous amount of information families throw our way. Third, in order to make use of this information, we need to look carefully at our own experience during exchanges with parents and how we act on that experience. For most helping professionals, however, this is easier said than done.

Many of us who work with parents were never taught to keep alive a running internal dialogue along the lines of "What do I feel now?" or "Is this experience unusual for me?" or "Am I acting in a way that expresses these feelings?"—in short, "How am I being transformed into reenacting the very problem the family needs to address?" The point of staying aware of our self-experience is to direct our advice in a way that helps people recognize just those taken-for-granted experiences (in psychologist Christopher Bolas's words, "the unthought knowns" [*The Shadow of the Object*, Columbia University Press, 1989]) that ultimately keep them stuck.

Becoming More Self-Aware

Over the years, I have found that staying aware of my own emotional states during contact with family members has uncovered at least three kinds of transformations particularly useful for directing interventions.

Embarrassing Emotions

The first category comprises transformations that are blatant and almost embarrassingly obvious. For example, Ed and Alice, a couple from New Jersey, came into counseling ostensibly because they were having disagreements about how to handle their preadolescent daughters. They also complained that they did not feel intimately connected to each other any more. During the first session, I was distracted from my usual line of questioning by strong sexual feelings toward Alice. This unsettling current of sexual electricity, atypical for me in a clinical setting, lasted for several meetings. In my embarrassment and consternation, I said nothing but took refuge in clinical technique—a kind of theoretical cold shower that got me through the sessions until the feelings passed.

Sometime later, Ed and Alice had almost stopped fighting and had improved their parenting skills. But they remained as emotionally unconnected to each other as when they came for the first interview. One day, Ed found a love letter to Alice from another man and discovered that she had been having an extramarital affair for most of the time they had been seeing me. In fact, during the beginning meetings, that seemed to me so sexually charged, Alice had begun a heavy flirtation with the man who eventually became her lover. At this point, Ed admitted to an ardent affair of his own 10 years earlier, a relationship so serious that when his lover suddenly ended it, Ed entered a period of mourning and disconnection from Alice that lasted for much of the decade.

With a jolt, I suddenly realized how I had been transformed to fit the particular contours of this couple's relationship. My intense sexual feelings, far from being a shameful distraction to be suppressed and ignored, had been a powerful clue to the secrets Ed and Alice were hiding. My lack of candor had made me not only a collusive silent partner in their mutual deception but a living enactment of the fundamental, unresolved issue in their marriage: dishonesty about intense emotions. A year later, their relationship had become far more turbulent and less civil, and they looked much more like a couple just beginning the hard, disrupting work of counseling. And I learned a lesson. By ignoring my own troubling internal experience, I had re-created their problem instead of challenging them to see it more clearly.

Obvious Emotions

Sexual feelings toward clients are unusual enough to make them recognizable as probable signs that we've become players in a family's drama. But the experience of other powerful emotional states isn't always such a clear-cut signal. Take anger, for example. When we are working with families, it is virtually impossible not to occasionally become outraged at the injustices going on between people in the name of love. Again, we usually try to think that harsh emotions from our coworkers, and even from ourselves, are "just life" and should be pushed away. But anger can sometimes burst forth with such surprising intensity that it can't (and shouldn't) be ignored. More often than not, we realize these feelings represent something other than momentary frustration, fatigue, or our own personal issues. Rather than being signs of our human fallibility, experiences of anger may be vital pieces of information about important but unacknowledged dynamics in the families who approach us.

One colleague, for example, a school counselor known for her gentle and courteous style, told me about a meeting with what she called "a family of barracudas and Philadelphia lawyers." "If one member of this family said one thing," she said, "another member aggressively refuted it. Everyone in the family, kids included, was constantly haggling and sniping at one another." Suddenly, this normally reserved professional found herself up to her neck in their fight: "I fell right into the soup, got enraged and started yelling as loudly as everyone else. One of the kids yelled back, 'Hey! I don't have to come here to get screamed at. I get enough of that at home!' "

This remark stunned the counselor simultaneously into awareness of what she was doing and triggered self-doubt. "What's come over me?" she wondered. "Maybe I don't have what it takes." She felt, in her words, that she had been "transformed" by this family, and she didn't fully recover her composure during the rest of the meeting. The next day she called the family to apologize for losing control, and the following week she said, "I've had a few days to think about what happened and how miserable it was for me to be arguing with you like that. It finally made me realize how awful it must be for you to go through that every day of your lives."

Immediately, the air cleared. The family relaxed and began to talk about how terrible and draining their arguments made them feel. Seeing someone who was "not them"—and a gentle person, to boot—become so volatile, and then miserable, painted an experiential picture impossible to ignore. For the first time, they did not simply take for granted or rationalize as normal the constant fighting in their lives. From that moment on, they were able to discuss their intrafamily struggles for power without reflexively blowing up at each other.

Now, I am not suggesting that we vent anger whenever the mood hits us or always share our experience. Nor do I believe that our errors are always diagnostically revealing. I am suggesting, however, that these errors can sometimes be vivid reenactments of exactly those issues most likely to be ignored, taken for granted, or off-limits for the family to address.

Subtle Transformations

Not all transformations that the counselor experiences in sessions are as dramatic and easily recognized as those involving anger and sexual arousal. But the following transformations, if uncharacteristic, offer sometimes dramatic clues about the people we see.

Repetitive Thoughts

Some are extremely subtle; they don't announce themselves in bold, emotional rushes, but hover on the edges of thought and feeling, where they are easily ignored. A young, unmarried couple, Ken and Diane, came to see me because Diane wanted greater commitment from Ken—marriage and a baby—while he was hesitant, unsure, and ambivalent, though he could never make clear what exactly held him back. He knew he loved Diane, he said, but—and here his voice always trailed away. We explored their feelings about the situation without making much progress.

Between meetings, however, I noticed that whenever I pictured Ken, I would see, superimposed on his face, that of a colleague named Frank. No matter how hard I tried to see Ken in my mind's eye, I could only visualize Frank. This little peculiarity, flitting at the edge of consciousness, didn't seem very meaningful, and certainly held no connection for me to what was going on between this couple.

One day, I was speaking to a friend and Frank's name came up. "You know, don't you," my friend said casually, "he's always had a problem with lying?" Then I remembered how often I'd felt with Frank that he was not telling me the truth, and I wondered again at his face settling over Ken's in my imagination.

In the next meeting, I asked the couple, "Are you sure you're being entirely truthful with me? What could be going on that isn't being talked about?" There was the familiar long silence that often comes before a major revelation, and then Ken began to disclose his real reasons for not wanting to get married. He was "addicted to women," as he put it, and was secretly so promiscuous that he worried about accidentally calling Diane the name of one of his many sexual partners. At the same time, he had convinced himself that this addiction was in a separate category of his life and not really relevant to his problems with Diane. Diane herself was noticeably unsurprised by this confession. "I had the sense that something was going on," she said, "but I always pushed it out of my mind. I didn't trust my intuition." Obviously, neither had I trusted mine. My difficulty remembering who was who, Frank or Ken, and dismissing the problem as trivial, perfectly enacted the most relevant and unspoken issue of this couple's life: Ken's deceptive habits and Diane's half-conscious, unarticulated recognition of the truth.

Our meetings, which had felt dead and pointless before, now took on new life. Ken initiated individual treatment in addition to the work with Diane. Eventually, after a long period of soul-searching, Diane decided to have a baby, with or without Ken's involvement. A baby—Ken and Diane's—was born a few years later. They still come in occasionally to discuss other issues of commitment and child rearing, but with the relevant matters out on the table, we are not continuing to act out a shadowy drama of pretense and deception (see the accompanying box).

Subtle Transformations to Be Aware Of

Many transformations are not quite so obvious. In fact, most of the important emotional and behavioral cues we can learn from are of what I call the subtle variety. Here are 10 of the most common transformations to notice. If any of them appear repeatedly during meetings with parents or children, ask yourself, "What underlying experience might this represent in these people?"

1. Calling a person repeatedly by the wrong name.
2. An unusual degree of boredom during meetings.
3. Doing personal mental business while trying to listen—laundry, shopping list, etc.
4. Giving one parent greater consideration than the other.
5. Being more validating and positive toward one.
6. Starting out sessions focusing on the same family member.
7. Asking questions of one parent more than his or her partner.
8. Being unusually brusque on the phone, overly solicitous, distracted, and so on.
9. How you end meetings: suddenly; go overtime; a friendly manner.
10. Being more sure of yourself or less so than usual.

Logistical Transformations

A second kind of subtle transformation is revealed in the way we set up the structure of meetings, whom we include (and don't), and especially how we handle money.

The Structure of Meetings

A striking example of this occurred when a colleague called me about a case he was supervising at his agency. The presenting problem was terrible fighting between elderly parents and their 24-year-old son, Luke. Luke was verbally abusive, took their money, and demanded that they give up any relationship that he could not directly monitor.

In this serious situation, my colleague acted in a way that was completely uncharacteristic. One of the most patient clinicians I have met, he advised his supervisee to deliver (in the second session) the following ultimatum: "I can't treat you together. I'll have to see you separately, because I don't think you should be living under the same roof."

When I reminded him of his usual patience, he said he was completely baffled by his own brusque advice, knowing that the ultimatum was impossible and essentially amounted to kicking the family out of treatment. Making impossible demands of one another was a pervasive way of life in this family, and now the supervisor—two steps removed—was reenacting this dynamic in the conditions he set for therapy. The family never returned. On the sidelines, we could only marvel at their power to transform not just the therapist but the "absent" supervisor as well.

Money Matters

The way professionals handle money is another transformational hot spot, often reenacting unspoken but crucial family dynamics. Over a decade ago I was working with a couple, Al and Karen, who had come in about fighting and Karen's increasingly serious depression. The couple's entire relationship was bound up in their family business. They spent all day together, Karen working as a secretary/

receptionist while also tending to the kids. Over the years she had become resentful and depressed. For his part, Al was angry over Karen's lack of appreciation for the "good deal" she was getting. Despite making progress with fights that could go on for weeks, Karen's depression did not lift and, if anything, became worse.

Believing that one of their difficulties was being under each other's skin all day—and feeling a little desperate—I found myself offering them a one-time-only opportunity: "If you join the local health club within 48 hours, I will give you a complete session of psychotherapy for free." I certainly knew my customers well, and at the next meeting they produced two Jack LaLane membership cards as coupons for a free session.

"A little quirky," I thought to myself, but at this stage of the game who was I to complain about any sign of improvement? And the health club did get them out of each other's hair, as well as improve their deteriorating physical conditions. Predictably, however, it didn't change their basic arrangement. Karen remained just as depressed.

Things began to move only after I went for a consultation. The supervisory team strongly recommended that Karen get a paying job outside the house. After the consultation, I understood the hidden meaning of my one-time-only offer. By reenacting the unexamined barter arrangement, I was trying to buy their health: if I gave my time away for free (just like Karen) and offered a "good deal to boot" (just like Al), things should improve. Fortunately for them, when things subsequently did not get better, I became worried enough to ask for help (see the accompanying box). Since the consultation, Karen has worked outside the house, which fundamentally shifted the power relationship. As a result, her depression has become more manageable, and the couple moved to Arizona in relative peace and harmony.

How to Recognize Transformations

The sooner we recognize that we have been transformed by parents or families into reenacting their most central dynamics, the more likely we are to know when and how to intervene effectively. It is

How You Handle Meetings, Money, and Other Logistical Matters

Sometimes transformations do not occur in the realm of emotional experience. Often, in fact, they pop up around issues that have to do with the logistics of our work. These include the way we handle money with people and the ways we set up meetings. These are often the first indicators of strong unaddressed issues that the family is triggering and that ought to be focused on in your work with them. Consider the answers to these questions:

1. To whom do you hand the bill?
2. Whom do you call for the parent–teacher conference?
3. Whom do you assume is responsible for arranging the conference?
4. Do you keep up with the client or the agency's collection system?
5. Did you set an unusually high or low fee for the meetings?
6. Have you been more or less available to a worried parent?
7. Whose schedule are meetings centered around?
8. Whose phone number do you use?
9. Who gets to sit in the more comfortable seat: do you offer a choice, or do they take turns?
10. Whom do you mostly talk to?

important to remember that no one is immune to this phenomenon. Whether you are a teacher, a counselor, case worker, or physician; whether you see people once a week or sporadically over the years; or whether there's a crisis and a parent asks for help—it is crucial to be aware of your own experiences and *use* them instead of ignoring or acting them out. Here's how:

1. Take a genogram. A genogram is another term for a family history. This is standard practice these days for many family therapists and should be used by anyone dealing with families.

For example, Ophelia, the mother of an obstreperous fifth grader, Anna, approached the teacher for advice about how to handle Anna's emotional outbursts. The teacher, Lenore, found herself as quickly aggravated with Ophelia as she was with her daughter. Lenore was just about to sharply reprimand Ophelia when she remembered the transformation phenomenon. Recognizing that her experience ought to be used as a guideline rather than ignored, Lenore asked Ophelia whether other people in her family have been prone to short fuses. She quickly took a family history and learned that, indeed, Anna's aunt, grandmother on Ophelia's side, and younger brother all had trouble containing their anger. This perspective helped Lenore temper her own judgments and allowed her to start helping Mom in a constructive way.

If you see a history of impulsivity in the family, you will not be so shocked when you find yourself tempted to impetuously reveal to your clients every thought, feeling, and bright idea you have about them.

2. Know your own responses. Knowing well our characteristic responses to different kinds of situations helps us recognize family issues that may trigger our own vulnerabilities.

To illustrate, a school counselor, the survivor of a family ravaged by the Holocaust, cannot trust her feelings of outrage when kids tease and abuse each other. Because of her history, this professional's judgmental stance toward any bully is a characteristic of her past and does not represent a transformation caused by a particular family or child.

Another example is a pediatrician I know who went through a terrible divorce. For the period of almost a year, he became easily outraged by "neglect" of mothers he met in his practice toward their children. Again, this was not so much a result of anything the mothers were actually doing to the kids but was an expression of his own experience going through a very troubling separation.

This kind of self-knowledge makes a powerful case for requiring family-of-origin coaching and consciousness-raising about race, gender definitions, and sexual orientation to be part of training. If this doesn't already exist, suggest it for your agency.

3. Be aware of everyday stresses and strains. These discomforts often make us subtly vulnerable to misreading what is going on. Fatigue, illness, an argument at home, financial pressures—all affect the way we view our clients. The unusual interventions we then try may not be reenactments of secret issues in the family but just bad judgment based on our own life difficulties.

For example, years ago, my 1-year-old daughter was sick with pneumonia. Though her temperature had stabilized and she was feeling better, I was still unsettled and anxious when I went back to work later in the day. That afternoon, I did a consultation with a very likable couple whose presenting problem—a history of drug abuse—was serious, but no more difficult than other cases I regularly take on. After listening to them for a while, I heard myself saying wearily, "I don't think I'm quite up to handling your problems, but I know a therapist who is much stronger in this area than I am."

I did refer them to a clinician more experienced than I with people in recovery from addictions, but on reflection I was struck by the way I had emphasized my weakness and incapacity, and how fragile I had felt during the session. In fact, for the entire day, I had been feeling like what I imagined my daughter to be—weak, vulnerable, exhausted—a first-time father viscerally identifying with his sick child. Unfortunately, I'm sure the couple left feeling not only rejected but convinced that their problem was a lot worse than they had thought.

Years ago, I saw the same phenomenon occur with a colleague of mine, Susan, who was working as a caseworker at a city agency. She had come to me for a consultation because she was getting into arguments with families about their misuse of money. After a few moments discussing her cases and recent events in her life, it became clear that Susan, who had recently been bumped in her Civil Service position to a lower salary, was vulnerable when it came to financial issues. It was Susan's own economic distress more than the actual behavior of the families that made her feel such outrage. Sure, some of her clients were not always responsible, but their behaviors did not merit the brunt of Susan's own anxiety about money.

These situations are legion, and they have less to do with the family's power to transform us than with the challenge of trying to work with people and live life at the same time. Only if we know ourselves—and recognize our characteristic responses to the ebb and flow of daily life—can we separate the transformations that are useful, trustworthy indicators of a family's problems from those emotional reactions that are based on our own personal difficulties.

Warning: Sharing of emotions with patients can be hazardous to your professional health. I do not recommend sharing of feelings with clients. As I suggested, use the emotional information to help guide your questions. Once the underlying issues in the family become clearer, emotional reactions usually settle down. If they don't, seek out a supervisory consultation or discuss in a peer support group.

*　　　*　　　*

Twenty-five years ago, my first supervisor regularly complimented trainees after sessions by saying, "So, you've worked yourself out of that mess pretty well." We thought he was reminding us that we had just managed to scrape by in spite of our obvious incompetence. Thousands of painful lessons later, I understand a little better what he meant. The "messes" we get ourselves into and work ourselves out of are those inevitable moments of transformation, recognition, and recovery that often are the deepest and most healing moments between ourselves and the people who come to us for advice.

Ironically, after decades of professionals helping *others* be more aware, the field's newest frontier may be a heightened respect for our own internal emotional experiences. And yet, perhaps it is not such a new step after all. The brilliance of the master therapists, teachers, physicians, and healers we've long observed on videotape emerged from trial-and-error mistakes based largely upon knowing exactly who they were and paying close attention to the emotional interplay between themselves and their patients, students, or clients. Unfortunately, their errors (and there must have been many) got left on the cutting-room floor. Now, as our understanding of the work changes, we can all be more mature. We can pick up those outtakes—those enlightening mistakes and fruitful errors—and make them part of a richer, more realistic vision of the helping relationship.

chapter
six **Staying in Charge**

Helping Parents Avoid the Traps
of Modern Parenthood

Helping parents take charge is an especially critical task for professionals these days. Most of
the parents and families I've interviewed express how pressed emotionally and physically families feel. Kids repeatedly mention this to
me in interviews and think a great deal about how vulnerable their
parents seem. In fact, as we've understood for decades, one of the
reasons children act out is to get that help for their parents—they
intuitively sense when the family is adrift and needs a firmer hand
on the tiller. Children feel better knowing that someone is taking
care of their parents, teaching them to become stronger and more
effective.

Yet, helping professionals have been surprisingly naive about
the many ways one can compassionately instill greater discipline.
Twenty years ago, when I was first being trained in family therapy,
the field was immersed in a celebration of therapeutic heroism. The
training tapes of the day popularized a variety of strong-arm tactics.
I remember the awe I felt while observing a 5-year-old disobedient
girl apparently "cured" after a stormy confrontation during which
her mother forced the girl to "sit still and listen" for 5 minutes. Another famous example showed the parents of a seriously anorexic
adolescent trying to stuff a hot dog down her throat; yet another
showed a disempowered father rising from his stupor to wrestle his
disrespectful teenage son to the floor. It was common to encourage

parents to drag their school-phobic kids off to class kicking and screaming. Some practitioners even went so far as to advise parents to disappear mysteriously for a few days, leaving a vague note for their chronically ill children concerning their whereabouts. For much of the field's history, family therapy's approach to establishing hierarchy has been much like 17th-century philosopher Thomas Hobbes's description of life: "nasty, brutish and short." Assert power over the kids quickly, in any way possible.

These techniques achieved popularity because they seemed to work and also because they represented an alternative to the limitations of Dr. Spock-inspired parental permissiveness, which many professionals who helped children welcomed. By the mid-1970s, the climate of opinion had grown more conservative. Social commentators frequently blamed liberal, easygoing, overindulgent child-rearing methods for producing the 1960s generation of hippies and rebels. More recently, we have begun to realize the problem with the premises underlying slam-bang approaches. First, these techniques assumed that a knowledge of child development doesn't matter: one intervention fits all ages. Second, it was assumed that making any dramatic change in a family automatically improved the level of parenting skills. Disciplinary problems, for example, were supposed to reflect dysfunctional marital patterns. Once the spouses had learned to deal better with each other, they had little to say about the basic skills necessary to keep a family running—from getting the kids up in the morning to putting them down at night, and everything in between.

In what follows, then, I am going to bring the theoretical and the practical together, a synthesis sorely missing in the training of child professionals. Whether it is teachers, guidance counselors, clergy, or camp counselors and directors, it is painfully clear to me that few have received any training in how to integrate abstract principles of child development with concrete parenting skills. With one eye toward child development and the other focused on problems of *modern* kids, I next suggest numbers of concrete ways you, the child professional, can help parents be more in charge of their children.

Creating Effective Consequences

From countless discussions I've had and seminars I've given, professionals who work with parents recognize the following fact of modern family life: it is almost impossible for many of today's parents to make clear to children what the *consequences* of their behavior will be. It's not that parents don't react to kids' indiscretions or defiance, they just don't create connections between a child's particular action and the consequences that follow. For example, in one family I saw, the kids were frequently rowdy at dinner, their rudeness escalating to pushing, punching, and under-the-table kicking. One evening, without warning and apparently without conscious thought, the mother, Margo, suddenly roared, "NO MOVIES FOR 2 MONTHS!" The kids looked at her in total disbelief, their sarcastic expressions saying plainer than words, "Yeah, right," and then resumed hostilities. To a child's concrete way of thinking, the consequence for the specific misbehavior—a movie embargo for fighting at the table—made absolutely no sense and was probably unenforceable anyway.

Many of us can relate to Margo's heartfelt but completely ineffective reaction. All manner of unenforceable threats and bad discipline habits take place daily in homes across America. So, from a variety of sources—parents, teachers, and children—I have compiled a half dozen of the most important principles that help parents to create consequences and stay in charge. As helping professionals our armamentarium needs to be expanded so that we can suggest concrete actions for parents to take. The following are phrased in ways that can be used by you with parents in many different situations:

1. Think before acting. Parents sometimes create consequences with little sense of their real feelings. Often, what pops out of parents' mouths is a reflex—a spasm of frustration and rage uninformed by what was *actually* bothering them. So, to help parents come up with more effective responses, I ask them two questions:

"What are you feeling during this interaction?" and "What, besides corporal punishment or running off into the night, would be the logical consequence of how you feel?"

In this case, Margo described how exhausting dinnertime monitoring was—especially after putting in 10- to 12-hour workdays. My question was, "If dinner makes you this tired, what would a logical alternative be?" Mom replied, "Give up dinners every night, and have family dinnertime just once a week. The other nights, we'll leave out food for the kids to prepare themselves."

Does this seem to be any kind of hardship for the children or even a real punishment? Of course not. But I am not simply interested in helping parents punish children. In place of parents' angry outbursts, I want to substitute an understanding of the connection between their behavior and its consequences. First, giving Margo a choice helped her take her own feelings seriously (which is crucial to effectively taking charge). Second, the suggestion to do away with a fundamental ritual of their family life stunned the kids into actually *hearing* Margo, instead of tuning her out. Did they become perfect dinner partners? No, not even close. But by helping herself feel less trapped in the nightly pandemonium, Margo had begun to take charge of a practice that had caused much grief.

In another, much more serious example, a 12-year-old boy and his 10-year-old sister were stealing from their parents—money, food, their parents' favorite clothing. No amount of screaming, lecturing, or hitting had worked. Recently, the two children had begun shoplifting around the neighborhood, which frightened the parents into seeking help. I asked Mom and Dad, "How does this make you feel?" "Like we're being violated," they replied. So, what's a logical response to violation? "Protect yourself." They decided to put locks on the doors and all the cupboards and to stop making ineffective speeches and threats.

Why would this suggestion have any effect? Might it not just make Mom and Dad feel like prisoners in their own home? Instead, to everyone's surprise, it brought a new sense of freedom to the parents and responsibility to the children. When the kids saw the locks on the doors, they knew for the first time that the adults were *serious,* and saw that doors and cupboards locked against them in their own home was the logical consequence to their petty theft. The 10-year-old actually approached Mom and said, "Gee, were we bothering you by taking your things?" For the first time they were able to talk about the conflict and come up with rules that made sense to both the parents and the kids.

In another example, Judy, a sixth-grade teacher, actually stopped "teaching" her class because of the incredible rudeness and disrespect she had been witnessing. Judy said to her students, "We have to go back to basics. I'm finding it impossible to teach when I'm so angry and hurt at the way you treat yourselves and me. So, for the next week I am going to teach basic respect in this classroom: not interrupting, not calling out, paying attention to the impact of what you say to everyone else." Judy's description of her own experience in the classroom was right on target. Her willingness to share her feelings and then create a logical consequence got the students' attention. In reviewing progress in her class at the end of the year, everyone involved—Judy, the guidance counselor, the students, and the parents alike—believed that this was the turning point to what was becoming an increasingly out-of-control situation.

2. Expect a counterreaction. Unfortunately, just because parents have changed *their* parts doesn't mean children aren't attached to the old script. Frequently, kids try to re-create the familiar scenario. Therefore, any time you ask parents to change the dance, prepare them for the child's *counterreaction.* For example, one child, Adam, was particularly creative in his efforts to get his father into the old game. When Dad walked away from a fight and closed his bedroom door rather than engaging in the familiar shouting match, Adam sat outside the room and bounced a rubber ball against the door more than a hundred times.

In almost every situation, kids don't simply roll over and *thank* Mom or Dad for their firmer, more thought-out consequences. Expect a challenge, and help parents be prepared. Help them to practice their planned response, and they will find it easier to endure their child's counterreaction.

3. Remain firm. Because we *had* prepared him, Dad stood firm, and Adam, this angry and rebellious 12-year-old, did something rather astonishing. He stopped throwing the ball and slipped a note under the door that read, "I'm sorry." Another kid whose parents remained firm during the counterreaction went outside and started throwing pebbles against his parents' bedroom window to get their attention. A 13-year-old girl actually walked to a pay phone and called home just to get a conversation going.

4. Ask kids what they think is an appropriate consequence. One apparently paradoxical approach to reestablishing a hierarchy is asking the children for their ideas about what might help. Even though kids are brought into the process, parents still retain the right to say no, thus keeping their place in the hierarchy. True, children may come up with crazy and unrealistic schemes—for example, "If I start studying more and pass, I should get a vacation to Hawaii." But often they think of surprisingly ingenious and workable solutions. For example, one boy's school performance was so bad that he was about to flunk out. His father, Henry, had spent most week nights and much energy alternately cajoling, reasoning, and yelling to get his son to do his homework. All with predictably negative results.

So, I encouraged Henry to ask the boy what he thought should be done. "Listen, Ernie, we've got a problem here," said Dad. "I'm bothering you every night because you won't do your homework, and it's driving me crazy. I want you to come up with a solution—and we'll consider it." Ernie's solution to the study problem was unexpectedly simple: "Let me do my homework in the kitchen, where everybody else is." It turned out that working alone at his desk, with no stimulation or people around, made him feel as if he were in an isolation chamber. Ernie knew what he needed, only somebody had to ask and then decide if it was appropriate—a basic way to increase parental power.

5. Provide a limited choice. Some children stubbornly resist any hierarchy. As described in Chapter 3, they are endowed with an excess of tenacity. Power struggles seem to consume most of the day. Luckily, we can provide a *limited choice*. This allows children to retain some autonomy while recognizing that they cannot put off the inevitable. The secret to effective limited choice is in the wording. For example, *"When* [not "if"] you clean up your room, do you want me to help or do you want to do it alone?" Whether the child decides one or the other is besides the point; it is a choice structured by the adult. Another way of saying this to parents is the following: "Offer your child two choices, *both* of which you can live with."

For example, Elizabeth, a 10-year-old girl who had been seriously anorexic for 1½ years, started to eat again when her parents insisted on these choices (listen to the structured options offered): "You can begin to eat here, with us, or in the hospital. And, you can increase your daily caloric intake by 200 per week or 400 every other week. Which do you choose?" When I saw the girl a couple of months later, I asked why she was finally eating. Her reply: "Because they seemed so sure of themselves that it was *out of my hands*. So, it won't be my fault if I get fat." With medication, brief family treatment, and her mother monitoring every single meal (Elizabeth chose to stay out of the hospital and increase her intake by 400 calories every other week), Elizabeth's obsession with food calmed down significantly enough after 3 months that she was able to resume her activities. This sudden turnaround is unusual, but the basic paradigm of providing limited choice is similarly effective for many situations.

6. Tie consequences to the next significant event in a child's life. This is especially helpful with kids who are old enough to have a developed sense of time—middle and high schoolers. Let's say a concert is coming up in 2 weeks. Use the concert as an immediate consequence, because that's what kids most want. The next event is usually where parents have true leverage. Kids begin to think, "Wait a minute—if I want to be able to go hang out on Friday night at Johnny's house and I don't do what they're asking me, I may not end up at Johnny's house." This concrete consequence tied to a real desire has way more leverage than any abstract lecture.

Alternative Ways to Create Consequences

Bribery

Modern parents are forbidden by all that is PC ("parentally correct") to use many old-fashioned parenting stratagems because they seem oppressive and are assumed to permanently warp the child's budding personality. One such myth of modern child rearing is that bribery is a corrupt and unethical way of gaining compliance and will probably turn the child into a future con artist. I started questioning this notion when the mother of two defiant preteens got them to come to a session by allowing the kids to roller-skate to the clinic. I was also humbled when my own child was 3 years old and, out of desperation, I floated an Oreo cookie on a boat in the middle of the tub in order to get her to take a bath.

The fact is that although bribery is out of fashion, nobody around today could have grown to reasonable adulthood (or will survive parenthood) without it. But whether it is called a "reward," an "incentive," or an "inducement," parents need to use bribery *well* to get anything done. Bribery becomes a problem when it is the *only* tactic parents have for getting their kids to listen to them. At that point, bribery by parents turns into extortion and the house has been taken over by the kids. Bribery also has a disturbing sound because in our consumerist culture we tend to think of it in exclusively materialist terms, as a kind of booty in money or clothes or a new pair of roller blades. In fact, there are other, more effective incentives for children. The following are some typical and alternative forms of consequences:

1. By all means, use material bribery. Parents and teachers should not be above using as rewards the "stuff" kids crave in return for desired behavior. Tried-and-true stickers, contracts, and verbal agreements should be a part of every parent's armamentarium and every teacher's classroom: "If you go 3 days in preschool (or grade school) without hitting another child, we'll give you 5 stickers. When you collect 20, you'll get that action figure from

Star Wars." These out-and-out rewards are absolutely essential in the real-life terrain of everyday living.

2. Use sequential rewards. Sequential rewards are often more palatable to parents, because they smack less of outright bribery to them. Sequential rewards are those little agreements we make with kids to keep the day running more smoothly. Remember this conceptual phrase when advising: *"If a child does _____, then he can _____."* Kids of all ages understand the "If–then" mode of discipline because they also want to get to the next activity. So, use sequential rewards to build parental leverage naturally and unobtrusively into daily life: "If you put your clothes on now, you can watch a few minutes of 'Hey, Arnold,' " or "If you stop playing in 5 minutes, we'll have more time to read together."

3. Offer one-on-one time as an effective incentive. Giving children solo time and attention with their parents is a reward that superbly fits our pressure-cooker world. It is often worth 100 video games to kids, who want their parents' precious attention more than anything else. In discussions with thousands of families and interviews with hundreds of kids, the resounding conclusion was that one-on- one time with parents is the best possible incentive to good behavior. Even 15 minutes a night without siblings around can create powerful and effective leverage, regardless of a child's age. It is important, however, that parents consistently follow through and spend the promised time with their children, and do soon after it's promised so that the reward remains connected to the behavior. Maria, a particularly resourceful single mother I met years ago in Brooklyn, would take each kid on the bus for an hour's ride, just the two of them. Her kids deeply valued these excursions, and they would rarely risk displeasing her and having the privilege withdrawn. Besides being a wonderful, relaxed means of parent–child connection, the bus rides were a highly effective source of leverage and maintaining control.

4. Use altruism to gain greater leverage. Another indirect but extremely powerful incentive to good behavior is parents' requesting help from their kids (especially preteens and adolescents) in some area that taps the child's special expertise. Parents can get the most recalcitrant, morose teenager to become helpful and (temporarily) affable by asking, "Would you help me repaint the basement [or fix this computer glitch, or pick out an outfit I can wear to the office party]?"

5. Actions speak louder than words. Sometimes actions teach more effectively than words, rewards or any technique. A while back someone told me about a now apocryphal story in which the writer described a highly effective way his father created an unusual but powerful consequence. The boy and his adolescent friends had damaged a house in a summer bungalow colony. His father and the other dads came back and saw the damage. His buddies got yelled at, publicly shamed or hit. His own father looked at him, didn't say a word, and left the scene. He came back an hour later with a stack of wood tied to the top of the car. All night long, Dad rebuilt the house that the kids had damaged. The writer said his father taught him more in that one night *by his actions* than any corporal punishment or heavy-duty consequence could have: the need to concretely make up for wrongdoings.

Guilt

Guilt has also gotten a bad name in modern child-rearing circles. Evoking images of damaged "adult" children recovering from their "toxic" childhoods, many parents have sworn off the use of guilt. Yet, used sparingly, it is a necessary and highly effective means to get through to today's kids.

1. Don't be afraid to cry. High on the list of unacceptable reactions is a show of impotence. Yet, this is sometimes precisely what gets through to the most ornery kids. For parents trying to stay in charge, the discretionary use of guilt is a powerful way of showing kids the impact of their actions. For example, Amy, the single mother of three kids, had been unemployed for several years and scheduled for a job interview the next day. She was extremely nervous. That evening, her children badgered her mercilessly for new high-tech sneakers, a luxury she could hardly afford. Amy tried every modern and old-fashioned parenting technique she knew—rational discussion, reproach, stern orders, hysterical threats, yelling—but nothing worked. Suddenly, she began to cry, saying to her kids: "I really need your help now. I'm so nervous I can't stand it. You've got to help me in some way." This unexpected move broke the war of nerves. Her 11-year-old stopped his badgering and said, "Are you upset, Mom?" Fifteen minutes later, this ordinarily sullen preteen came back with a "happy" rainbow card he had made for her.

2. Express all those unparent-like emotions. Between the ways we behave *and* the two-dimensional portraits of mothers and fathers in the popular culture, it's hard for kids to remember that parents are three-dimensional people with feelings too. Professionals often don't realize how important it is to help parents express more emotion than just anger and frustration. There are many other emotional "colors" to child rearing that parents feel are "unparentlike" to express to their children: hurt, disappointment, feeling left out, rejected, anxious—a whole range of human experience that parents don't express because they believe they're not supposed to.

Again, if parents rely too often on emotional displays, they become ineffective. Kids, like adults, grow cynical in the face of repeated shows of martyrdom aimed at gaining some advantage over them. But an atmosphere of emotional honesty teaches children that what they do sometimes makes other people suffer—a revelation that startles them. Because of this, I often ask parents to once or twice a week express "unparentlike" emotions that convey their humanity (e.g., "I feel hurt when you do that," "I'm scared," "I need you," or "I'm disappointed"). Far from undermining authority, such admissions strengthen children's awareness of their impact on others, make them experience a sense of remorse for hurting other people, and lessen their ability to tune out their parents' needs.

For example, Pearl, with some accuracy, called herself a doormat. She came to me because Billie, her son, didn't listen to teachers, to friends, or to her at home. One day, after discussing together how his dismissive, arrogant attitude made her feel, Pearl went shopping with him. Billie threw a fit because Mom needed him to go for a minute or two to help her get something photocopied—for *herself.* Pearl reported to me: "You know what? I finally saw how hurt and abused I often feel. So I said to him, 'You're really hurting my feelings, all the time I do things for you, and you literally won't spend two minutes to help me out!' " Pearl admitted, "It was hard for me to say that. I thought I was laying guilt on him. But you know what? All of a sudden Billie 'got it.' He looked at me and said, 'You mean getting that stuff copied really matters to you?'" "Yes," Pearl said, "*my* feelings count too!" From that moment Pearl began to pay attention to her own emotional responses. These proved to be accurate signals of when Billie was stepping too far out of line—way before she exploded or he got into serious trouble.

Read Parents Their Rights

In order for modern parents to stay in charge, it is necessary to remind them of their rights as grown-ups. In our upside-down culture driven by the "second family" (see Chapter 7), trendmakers, and pop psychologists, we often forget how unempowered many parents feel. So, when it comes to staying in charge, they need to be "read their rights." Here are the most important:

1. You have the right to change your mind. If you think about it, parents create consequences that are absolutely unenforceable: they come out in a moment of anger; they make no sense to anyone (including us) after we make them. Yet, we've all worked with mothers and fathers who are afraid to change positions because it would be inconsistent.

Fear of inconsistency—the appearance of waffling—is another myth of modern parenting practice. In fact, the opposite message, "We adults think about things and will change our minds if we believe it's appropriate," suggests to kids that parents are in control of themselves. For example, a divorced dad found himself locked in a particularly torturous punishment *he'd* laid down—sitting by his teenager's side for 3 days straight until the boy had rewritten a plagiarized term paper. Dad felt more beleaguered than his son but was paralyzed about being inconsistent until I encouraged him to say, "Listen, I was thinking about this monitoring idea, and it's off base. I'm going to change it to the following: I'll be in my room doing my own stuff. After you've finished each section, come and show it to me." Far from creating more insolence, this thoughtful about-face strengthened Dad's position. He suddenly realized that nothing was written in stone and became more flexible and confident about his decisions.

2. You have the right to slow down the action. Fast-talking kids use pressure tactics to get immediate permission for something that would probably appall most parents—if they had the time to find out what was really on their kids' minds. This becomes a serious problem as children grow older. Almost all preteen and teen parties that involve the use of drugs or alcohol are organized at the last minute by kids saying to their befuddled parents, "I've got to know *now!*" Parents in this position should respond, "No, you can't go. If you want to go next time, you'll have to ask me sooner." Prepare for a major counterreaction here; but last-minute pressure tactics are not a healthy way for a parent to make smart decisions.

3. You have the right to call other parents. Across all economic and social groups, parents say that kids are outraged if they want to get in touch with other parents. These days, parents feel like hostages to threats such as "I'll never trust you and tell you anything again," or they worry that "The kids will feel betrayed and will hate us forever." If you assume that, deep down, kids really want to be in charge of adults, this is true. But if you believe, as family therapist Marianne Walters has written, that kids need us to be "strong and sure," then their outrage usually gives way to relief.

A particularly vivid example was 16-year-old Megan, whose parents asked me whether they should allow her to go to an unchaperoned all-night party after the high school prom. Megan had been incensed when her parents requested that they be "allowed" to call other parents, predictably saying that "All the other parents are letting *their* kids go to the party." With my encouragement, Megan's mom finally did call and discovered that, in fact, *none of* the other parents even knew of the party's existence. After her initial outrage and sense of betrayal subsided, Megan told me privately that she had been relieved when her parents put their foot down and "took her off the hook."

When Your Suggestions Fail

It is sometimes impossible for families to create reasonable consequences even after we professionals intervene. However, the most valuable change often happens as a result of the failure of our parenting suggestions. Here's how to snatch victory from the jaws of defeat.

1. **Use a mental checklist.** If a few weeks go by with no noticeable changes, ask yourself the questions listed in the accompanying box.

2. **Look for family-of-origin dynamics.** If you've checked out these questions, the most likely explanation is an unaddressed family-of-origin issue. As I've indicated, generations-old issues often explode around failed advice. This forces to the surface hidden issues that have long kept parents ineffective.

For example, a 7-year-old girl, Lilly, had an eating disorder and was derisive toward her mom, Helen, even to the point of being actively abusive toward her. I said to Helen, "Listen, when she curses at you, walk away. See if you can go to your room, lock the door, and calm yourself down." For weeks, Helen failed each time, expressing concern that such a sharp dismissal of her daughter would emotionally damage the child. I asked, "Is separating, even for short periods, viewed as dangerous in your family of origin?" Mom replied, "Well, sometimes I have a hard time not answering my

Consequences Checklist

1. Was I expecting too much?
2. Did the kids "get" what was expected?
3. Did Mom or Dad understand my advice?
4. Did they actually agree to try it?
5. Should we search together for a less demanding change?
6. Was it the right advice, or did I miss the boat?
7. Is there a personal demon or family secret operating here?
8. What family beliefs make my advice impractical?
9. Did we prepare well enough for the kids' counterreaction?
10. Is it really a question of appropriate consequences, or does the child suffer from some underlying disorder (see Chapter 2)?

phone because I'm afraid it's my mother and something might be wrong with her." It was quite a bit of high drama when Helen was finally able to say "Listen, Mom, I'm not going to pick up every call that comes in, even if it's you. Sometimes I'm just too busy." Shortly after this move, Helen began taking 2 hours every Saturday morning "to run errands for myself." Helen was soon able to walk away when Lilly was in midtantrum and finally take a firmer hand in her daughter's discipline.

3. When you're stuck, open up the system. This is a fancy way of trying to find a previously hidden ally for a beleaguered parent. Start searching anywhere in the family—taking a genogram is helpful. Be creative: sometimes you'll find an ally with the parents of a boyfriend or girlfriend; get those two families together.

For example, 12-year-old Olivia had been getting into terrible fights with her mom, Candace. The two seemed unable to lower the degree of intensity and rage between them. Candace was beside herself, especially after unsuccessfully trying numbers of parenting techniques. Feeling stuck, we drew a genogram and I asked Candace if anyone else in the extended family could serve as a substitute Mom for the next couple of days. Candace has a younger sister, Micki, whom she believed would be less susceptible to Olivia's provocations. After discussing the issue thoroughly with Micki, including ways of staying in touch, Candace suggested that Olivia take a break and spend the night with her aunt. Opening up the system like this is often the most expedient and effective way of helping parents and kids get out of recurring and seemingly intractable dances.

Helping parents actively resolve family-of-origin issues can clear the way for them to use new parenting options that had previously failed. Many parents, of course, come to child professionals with no interest whatsoever in exploring their families of origin. They just want to "get the kids in line." But when they get stuck and cannot implement simple child-rearing techniques, they begin to ask, "Why?" At this point, leftover family matters become relevant. And, with a bit of encouragement, many mothers and fathers become motivated to actively resolve the issues that prevent them from taking charge of their kids.

Compassionate Discipline: A Summary of Techniques to Create Effective Consequences

I include this glossary of consequences in almost every talk I give. When working with parents, use these guidelines as a reference to help them stay in charge. The techniques are organized according to developmental level.

Ages 2 to 5

- **Distract.** Rule of thumb: The earlier you intervene before bad behavior occurs and the more attention-getting the distraction, the greater your chance of success. Never try to distract a child in the throes of a tantrum; try to intervene earlier because, as family communication research shows, out-of-control behavior quickly escalates beyond distraction. Your child will immediately feel comforted when an adult is in charge of such a situation.

• **See tantrums clearly.** Learn to differentiate manipulative tantrums, which you should ignore, and temperamental tantrums, which occur when a child is ill, tired, hungry, or overstimulated and which should be tended to immediately.

• **Remove your child from a difficult situation.** A change of context often releases parent and child from feeling locked in battle.

• **Restrain your child from hurting himself or others.** A bear hug is very effective as you say, "I won't let you hit again." If he screams and squirms, hold tighter. When he feels your conviction, he'll stop.

• **Use *brief* time-outs.** Remember to use short, enforceable periods and send your child to a quiet place—without entertainment. Don't add to the struggle by suggesting, "Think about what you did wrong." Explain in a *brief* sentence why you've done it ("I can't think straight when you yell like that"). Calm yourself in the meantime.

• **Build sequential rewards into everyday routine.** Natural ways to get things moving, such as "If you get dressed more quickly, you can watch 15 minutes more of 'Barney,' " make the notion of rewards less arbitrary.

Ages 6 to 8

• **Offer sequential rewards—and negotiate.** Suggest a trade-off, such as "If you put on your socks now, then you'll have 5 minutes later for *Pokémon*." Don't expect immediate compliance to the first "deal" you offer—these children already like to bargain, and they'll try to expand 5 minutes to 10.

• **Offer limited choices.** "You can wash your face first or brush you teeth—which will it be?"

• **Leave a situation once it gets too hot.** Refuse to engage when your child utters that time-worn favorite, "It's not fair." (When you stop the escalation ["We'll talk about this later when we all calm down"], your child learns three important lessons: that there are good times and bad times to talk, that there are consequences to behavior, and that there are limits to how much she can challenge your—or any adult's—reserve of patience.)

• **Ask your child for solutions.** Grade school kids are hungry to take on more responsibility. It lets them know that you don't have all the answers and that you can work together. Their suggestions also give you a glimpse into their world—what they've picked up from the media and from friends.

• **Use an old-fashioned star system of rewards.** A child of this age appreciates structure and systems. But this strategy has a short shelf life, especially if it's overused. Best to do it with a specific goal—chores leading up to a particular reward.

• **Post schedules and lists of chores.** Like the star system, this is highly visible, systematic, and concrete. Let your child have input into which chores he does and the order in which he does them. This method seems less arbitrary to a child than expectations that come out of nowhere.

• **Use hypothetical situations to problem-solve.** For example, "Myra has trouble sharing toys. How do you think her parents can help her?" Or use TV characters or book plots as a springboard for a talk. Don't bring the lesson back to your child ("How do you think Myra's situation applies to you?").

• **Appeal to your child's sense of empathy.** Occasionally, be direct about your own feelings: "It doesn't seem fair when you talk to me like that. You wouldn't like it." This is a far cry from a rigid "Do-it-because-I-said-so" approach.

Ages 9 to 11

• **Put a time limit on all negotiations.** Tell your child, "We'll give you 5 minutes to prepare your best case; then we'll make a decision." Preteens love the art of the deal—they can easily wear parents down.

• **Make specific contracts.** Say, "If you come home at 4:00 [as opposed to "on time"] from your friend's house Monday through Thursday [versus "most of the week"], then you'll be able to stay out until 5:00 [versus "a little longer"] on Friday afternoon." Specificity leaves little room for interpretation or renegotiations.

• **Ask for solutions, but be prepared for the outlandish:** "If I clean my room, can I watch TV all day on Sunday?" It helps to remember that kids love negotiating more than the privilege or object they're asking for. This insight lets you calm down and gain a new perspective on the issue ("Tomorrow, she won't feel so bereft about not going to that party").

• **Respect your child's moodiness after a confrontation or when you've laid down a law he doesn't like.** Also, keep in mind your child's temperament. Such timing and sensitivity repeatedly tells your child that you understand who he is.

• **Try to forget "the room."** Close the door so you don't see the mess. If the bedroom threatens the rest of the house—an odor or insect infestation—then draw the line by giving your child a limited choice: "You can either clean it up on your own by tomorrow or we'll do it together [or I'll pay your sister out of your allowance to help me]." This lets a child know you won't automatically encroach on her territory—but since she lives with others, she must avoid encroachment on *their* territory.

• **Expanded privileges need to be earned; they are not inalienable rights.** This is the gateway to adolescence. Since preteens are more than capable of empathy during a calm moment, link your experience with their increasing freedom: "You can take the bus by yourself if you're home by 5:00. That way, I'll see that you can handle yourself, and I won't worry so much."

Ages 12 to 15

• **Write longer-term contracts.** You might suggest, "If you maintain a B average, you can take riding lessons next semester." Since most young adolescents think of any parental demand as a form of oppression, contracts help make the rules seem less emotionally charged. Allow a teen's input, but be sure he knows that you have the last word.

• **Pick your battles wisely.** With a teen, there are endless opportunities for conflict and, at the same time, increasingly powerful pulls from the peer group and pop culture. (The more you clash, the more she perceives the adult world as alien and stifling.) So, it might be wise to concede on a wild hairstyle while holding the line on curfew.

• **Be sure all consequences reflect these three points, which set limits and yet recognize your child's growing independence:**

1. State exactly what you want ("I don't want you smoking at the concert").
2. State what will happen if you find out he didn't comply ("I won't trust you and will end up worrying, so no more concerts for 3 months").
3. Acknowledge that you won't be there to monitor her ("In the end, you'll have to make your own decision, knowing exactly what I think and what will happen if you don't' listen").

Although teens are on the cusp of adulthood, the distance between two points will never be greater than at this age. However, these three steps send a rational message: while there are limits, we can't realistically enforce them all.

*   *   *

Most parents *want* to do the right thing—to connect more effectively with their children, which means to love and enjoy them, while also helping them become self-reliant and responsible adults. Establishing an appropriate hierarchy in the family is an essential way of *connecting* with our children. When they test the limits, they dare us to love them in spite of their worst selves and implicitly appeal to us to set boundaries that let them know they are safe and secure. Most mothers and fathers want to live up to this challenge but many need lessons in the concrete details of putting it into daily practice with their own children.

chapter seven — The Second Family

Working with Adolescents in a Dangerous World

Most helping professionals get so involved with the kids and families we meet we sometimes miss the social changes that are happening all around us. Every few years I encourage myself and other professionals to step back and take a look at the larger picture. The following chapter is the result of a review of hundreds of families I've met during the last decade. Usually I know it's time for such a review when I feel the work is simply getting too hard to manage. When it comes to adolescents, a regular review is almost mandatory, especially since their situation is increasingly more extreme.

Few professionals who work with adolescents have not commented on how much more difficult it is for today's kids to simply survive. Having supervised hundreds of counselors, school psychologists, group home leaders, and school teachers throughout the country, several years ago it became clear to me that a major change in the lives of adolescents was taking place. This realization was not sudden, but a cumulative learning experience from working with increasing numbers of teenagers who engage in risky behaviors.

For example, when his family was referred to me, 13½-year-old Jimmy was on the verge of being expelled from eighth grade because of his obvious but heatedly denied pot-smoking habit. Almost worse, according to his horrified parents, he intended to have his ears, eyebrows, and lips all pierced and various items of punk jewelry inserted. Jimmy's parents seemed to agree with his various therapists and counselors: The boy's problems, they had all said, could be traced to a distant father and an overindulgent and intrusive mother. Together, they had not set enough rules and limits for the boy's behavior. In short, Jimmy suffered from a basic inadequacy in the family hierarchy. Jimmy's father acknowledged that he had not had much of a relationship with his son since the boy's early childhood, and his mother admitted that he had been "emotionally spoiled"—she had gone back to work when he was a toddler and was always guiltily trying to make up for lost time with him. When Jimmy was a young child, Mom said, he used to confide in her, but, since the age of 8 or 9, he had gradually been moving out of her orbit. During the last couple of years, she didn't think he'd said five words to her that weren't requests to buy him something, give him money, or grant a new privilege. When Jimmy and I met, he was pleasantly uncommunicative—neither loudly belligerent nor silently sullen. He answered questions politely but with maddening vagueness, as if he were talking to a slightly less intelligent life-form from a distant world.

Since Jimmy had grown disconnected from his parents some time ago, I asked who had been the significant adults in his life, his role models, confidants, friends, or advisers. It soon became obvious that Jimmy hadn't experienced any significant connection with a grown-up, including his parents, since middle childhood. Beginning in about the third or fourth grade, he had almost completely drifted away from the adult world into the closed society of the kid pop culture, communing mostly with his TV, Nintendo and Sega video games, CDs, and "action" comic books. Friends came to hang out—none of whom his parents truly knew.

The other therapists had been partially correct—there was no meaningful authority in Jimmy's family. More to the point, however, there was little significant connection in the family. Insidiously, without his parents quite noticing it, Jimmy had, over the years, been completely engulfed by a voracious, commercially driven youth culture. Beginning in preadolescence and certainly by now, the "second family" of his peers had, in fact, become his primary family, the one that really mattered to him.

Unquestionably, Jimmy's parents needed help—there were no rules in the family—but there was little they could do in the way of good parenting as long as they lived in such separate worlds. And of what use would typical interventions be when the fundamental assumption upon which they were based—the parents' central importance to the child's life—hadn't been true for quite some time?

When it comes to millions of kids like Jimmy, counseling has not kept pace with several decades of massive social upheaval. The world of an adolescent is now so powerfully defined by forces other than home—the peer network, pop culture, school, and neighborhood ethos—that working with the family alone is rarely powerful enough to effect change in the life of a troubled teenager. This second family of peers and pop culture has developed such force it is time to publicly acknowledge what many counselors have privately long understood. As we have entered the 21st century, there is compelling evidence of the need to significantly redefine how professionals work with adolescents and children.

The Fragmentation of the "First Family" at Home

Today, the disintegration of the first family, for decades bleakly apparent in urban populations, has finally become palpable at all socioeconomic levels. Trends begun in the 1970s have dissipated the gravitational force of the first family. Jimmy is not an unusual case. As we all recognize by now, divorce (50% of marriages), mobility (up to 20% of the population moves every year), and economic pressures that generally require both spouses to work ever-longer hours have undermined the old stability of the family. The "traditional" configuration of male breadwinner and wife at home fits only 11% of today's households (see "The Second Family," *The Family Therapy Networker*, May/June 1996). Time-squeezed parents even in intact, dual-earning families have few moments to spend with their children. While studies differ on the matter, Lester C. Thurow shocked the parenting world when he wrote in *The New York Times* (" 'Survival of the Fittest' Capitalism Destroying Traditional Family," September 10, 1995) that parents now spend 40 percent less time with their children than they did 30 years ago and 2 million children under 13 have no adult supervision either before or after school. As I describe in Chapter 10, even if Thurow's findings can be faulted, there is little question that the quality of time spent together has become, during the past few decades, more frenetic and splintered. Each person is engaged in his or her own computer, phone, TV, e-mail, errand, and after-hours homework or work world.

Furthermore, the family's informal support systems—the extended kin networks, church and community organizations, PTAs, and neighborhood ties that buttressed family life—have gradually disintegrated. For example, PTA membership since 1964 has fallen from 12 to 7 million ("The Second Family," *The Family Therapy Networker*, May/June 1996). And while Main Street—with its network of well-known shopkeepers and familiar customers greeting one another every day—is too often deserted and half boarded up, huge impersonal malls on the fringes of town are the real center of urban and suburban life in America.

Enter the Second Family

Into the void left by the withering away of adult community life has rushed the vast wave of adolescent peer groups and pop culture. Their influence has been hugely expanded and energized by a technological explosion that has proven its power to blast into every home. Two-year-old children, without developed language ability, can recite the McDonald's jingle; indeed, researchers have found that 18-month-old kids are already capable of brand-name recognition. And, despite what your friends may admit, the average high school graduate has spent 15,000 hours of his or her life in front of the TV, compared with only 11,000 hours spent in school ("The Second Family," *The Family Therapy Networker*, May/June 1996).

Today's child has more than likely already been pried out of the family long before adolescence by the grasping tentacles of the pop culture. At a time when external forces—peer groups and mass culture—are at least as powerful in defining the adolescent's world as the internal family system, the old primary family system has become a shadow of its former self, often exerting less pull on the teen's heart, mind, and hormones than the second family of the peer group. For professionals working with kids, the consequences of this shift are enormous; we can no longer focus only on the first family we meet. It isn't enough, it doesn't work, and it's time to admit it.

Getting Parents and Teens Reconnected

From this wider perspective, it would have been pointless to try to create hierarchy in Jimmy's primary family without first bridging the great divide between parents and peers. For this, body piercing seemed as good an issue as any. The idea of multiple flesh piercings on a 13-year-old disturbed me too, but I told Dad that, rather than ineffectively rant and rave, he should use this event to get to know his son better—to find out about Jimmy's world—and to begin establishing the kind of connection that might actually give him some protective influence over Jimmy's life.

So, Jimmy's father offered to join him on exploratory rounds of various body piercing establishments; Jimmy, of course, refused, but his father, with my coaching, quietly pointed out that it was his duty as a parent to make sure he did it somewhere safe and hygienic. After a period of sulky resistance, Jimmy relented and said—not without pride—that "if it mattered so much," he would show his father the whole piercing scene. During this rather unusual definition of "quality time," father and son eventually compromised on two relatively tasteful earrings in one ear. The piercing was done at a respectable shop using fully sterilized implements.

This foray into Jimmy's world did not end the boy's problems by any means. But it both rekindled Dad's interest in parenting—he had been hurt and deeply demoralized by his son's rebuff—and set the stage for further rapprochement. Because Jimmy had a hard time getting to sleep at night, I suggested that his father sit with him for just a few minutes each evening. Over the course of several weeks, Jimmy began, for the first time in 10 years, to talk about his life—about his girlfriend, his troubles concentrating in class, and his best friend's abusive father. One day, he finally admitted the obvious—he was "experimenting" with pot.

After 3 months of these gradually unfolding efforts at connecting with his son, the father had built a sufficient relationship and the mother had let go of her resentments about being the only caretaker in the family. Only now could they adequately support a workable family hierarchy. When a fight erupted because Jimmy was not keeping curfew, his father and mother had both earned sufficient parental authority to successfully demand that it was time for him to see a drug counselor.

Helping Professionals
Learn about the Second Family

Most professionals are at a loss to understand the makeup and characteristics of the second family. Here are the main aspects they should know:

First, not only is the second family of today's peer and youth culture at least as influential as the primary family in the adolescent's life, it is likely to be just as dysfunctional. Consider the values expressed in the universal role models and fads of pop culture: anorexically thin teenage fashion models, endless consumerism, hypersexualized and violence-saturated entertainment, and an ethic of sophisticated hipness that makes kids seem old in spite of their obvious immaturity.

Second, since the peer group is essentially rudderless, it exemplifies Murray Bowen's concept of the "undifferentiated ego mass." Once in the group, individuals are not permitted to be fully themselves. They are implicitly forbidden, under pain of ostracism, to develop their own independent interests and values; if the old family hierarchy kept adolescents from ever leaving home, the new second family discourages them from going home, or going anywhere else away from the pack.

Finally, like the alcoholic or abusive parent who controls a dysfunctional family, so the teen leader—often one of the most disturbed kids in the group—sets the mores and behavior patterns for the rest. This is, of course, nothing new. Young people have always admired and emulated charismatic group leaders. But today the stakes are much higher. Instead of showing other kids how to inhale cigarettes, a 13-year-old might be introducing them to smoking pot and now, increasingly, smoking heroin; instead of making fun of an unpopular teacher, a 15-year-old with learning disabilities will use his charm and verbal wit to get other kids to spend the night spray-painting graffiti on the sides of the school building or engage in life-threatening sexual behavior.

How Professionals and Parents Can Intervene with the Second Family

If professionals are at a loss in terms of understanding the second family, they are even more paralyzed when it comes to taking action. We have not been trained to deal with the second family and don't quite know how to approach it. Here are some ways:

1. Find out who belongs. Usually, counselors and teachers will not see the charismatic dysfunctional leader of the peer group but another less socially skilled adolescent who gets "busted" for the activities of the second family. In these cases, it may be critical that the counselor not only take into account the second family but actually begin talking with those "family members," including the leaders. The question is, how? I often find out who my teenage clients' friends are because I ask every child I see (first grade and up) to draw a sociogram—the social equivalent of a genogram—of their peer group. This identifies second-family members and lets me know something about their influence as well as the kinds of problems they are having in their own lives.

2. Ask other second family members in. Some years ago, before I really understood the power of the peer group, I began to see 15-year-old Peter, whose history included shoplifting, selling drugs, and fighting over graffiti turf. After including his parents in counseling for a few meetings, I saw Peter alone. Actually he didn't come by himself but always brought along his buddy Kevin, who sat patiently in my waiting room during each session. Several weeks later, it suddenly dawned on me that Kevin was behaving much like the parent of any troubled child seeing a therapist. Might this be a way of announcing his own relationship to Peter, as another family member who also needed help?

One day, I asked Kevin if he would like to come in also. "OK," he said, without hesitating, then walked in, sat down, and began talking about his own truly terrible problems. He lived with a single, alcoholic mother who brought different men home with her. Kevin said he often stayed out all night because he was repulsed about going home. Peter seemed relieved that someone else besides him knew about Kevin's bad situation. After seeing this small "family" of two for several weeks, I encouraged Kevin, a chronic substance abuser himself, to come clean with his parents and join a drug program. (*Note: To find out whether or not you must advise the parents before seeing a child's friend, check your state requirements.*)

As always, changes in one part of a system can have a pronounced ripple effect. When Kevin stopped using drugs, so did Peter; after Peter quit, so did his girlfriend. With these barriers down, Peter later could move closer to his parents, revealing to them for the first time how far into chaos his life had drifted.

Now more alert to second-family dynamics, when I began seeing Julia, a 14-year-old girl with bulimia, I asked her if she would like to invite her best friend, Laurie, to visit for a couple of meetings. She was glad to. (*Note: Whether you work in a clinic setting or privately, if you plan to see a second-family member for more than one or two meetings, it's important to get the parents' permission, since they may be paying for the treatment.*) While Julia was withdrawn, secretive, and shy, Laurie was gregarious and talkative, a natural leader. Actually, however, Laurie was in more serious trouble than her friend, with multiple sexual partners and caught in the middle of a savage custody battle between her separating parents. It was obvious, too, that Julia was actually taking care of Laurie—acting as confidante, even receptacle, of Laurie's insatiable need to spill her guts.

Two weeks later, when Laurie's mask of bravado cracked, she asked if I could help her. After several phone calls to her parents emphasizing the truly perilous state of their daughter's situation, I persuaded them to enter divorce mediation rather than battling it out via lawyers. Once Laurie's parents had moderated their hostilities, she felt less frantic and could begin to put some emotional energy into improving her own life—drinking and sleeping around less, and attending a support group for girls with eating disorders. Because I had taken Laurie's problems seriously and freed Julia from the burden of saving her friend, Julia began to trust me and started talking more freely about her own difficulties.

3. Find out who the second family's leader is. To cross rigid peer group boundaries, counselors often must get permission from an important second-family member. Sometimes neither the rigidity of the boundary nor the identity of the key peer group member is immediately apparent. We're easily duped because most media-obsessed kids are highly sophisticated users of pop psychology. They've seen hundreds of therapists, counselors, and assorted mental-health gurus on TV, and can easily pass an hour glibly talking and "relating" without saying anything at all. Jared, for example, a 15-year-old with no connection of any importance to an adult, was ordered into drug counseling at his school, as a condition of probation. As is often the case, the counselor, Erica, thought everything was going well: Jared was polite and agreeable. And, though he didn't actually tell her much, she felt hopeful that once they "connected," he would open up—until he suddenly dropped therapy without warning or explanation.

Several months later, caught smoking marijuana, Jared was once more forced into counseling. At this point, Erica asked my advice and I suggested she call his girlfriend, Jenny, treating her exactly as if she were a family member whose permission and cooperation were needed for counseling to continue. As the counselor soon found out, Jared and Jenny were absolute soul mates—mutual caretakers and protectors, best friends, lovers, quasi-siblings. Jenny had been deeply jealous of and anxious about Jared's first therapist; she could not tolerate an adult female's getting close to him.

But, on the second try, when Erica asked Jenny for her "permission" to see Jared, showing her the respect she deserved as the person most central in Jared's life, Jenny lost her defensiveness. Holding Jared's hand, she told Erica how Jared, who seemed exceptionally smooth and self-confident, was often so lonely at night that he could not sleep and turned to pot for relief. So that they might both cut down on pot smoking, Jenny said, she had taken to calling him every night and talking until they dropped off with the phones in their hands.

Jared is still struggling with his drug problem and some long-ignored learning difficulties. But he has accepted his parents' idea of random drug testing as a way to keep himself on track—a major step for someone who had lived his life in secretiveness and hiding. Both he and Jenny are less isolated in the closed little world of each other's company; they are talking more openly to their parents and beginning to experience themselves as individuals, separate from each other.

Encouraging Parents to Reach Out to Other Parents

Many of today's parents feel that they stand alone, trying to hold on to their kids in a vast undertow that inexorably drags youngsters under and away. And compared to previous generations, they do stand alone. Mothers and fathers are certainly less likely to know the parents of their children's friends than they used to be. Far fewer adults engage in school activities (keep in mind the decline of PTA membership), and the school itself is more likely to be a huge centralized learning factory located some distance from many of the areas that feed it. But if parents are separated by geography, unforgiving work schedules, a hodgepodge of custody arrangements, or simply an energy deficit for extracurricular activities, their kids operate under no such disability. In one quiet, suburban neighborhood, for example, about a half-dozen 9-year-old boys were sneaking into a neighbor's basement after midnight and watching pornographic films. What struck me was that every fourth grader in the school knew about this after-hours cinema club. But when parents finally caught on, it took several days for the word to spread among them.

Or consider "raves" and loft parties, popular forms of adolescent dance events throughout the country. With no adults permitted, they often start at midnight and continue into the wee hours of the morning. These events make alcohol and drugs freely available to hundreds of mostly unacquainted teens. When the panic-stricken parents of a 13-year-old came to me about how to handle an upcoming loft party, it was shocking that not one other set of parents knew about it. Again, just about every kid in school knew the details and was plotting how to go.

If they want to regain any control before a crisis, mothers and fathers need to have some basic knowledge about their kids' lives. Like it or not, parents won't get the information they need without establishing some form of mutual intelligence system to compensate for the toss of traditional adult community. It is increasingly important that all professionals who work with children move out of the consultation room and into people's lives. For example, many teachers I know are getting involved in peer groups for parents. They meet with mothers and fathers every couple of months to find out what is going on at home and in the neighborhood. School counselors are initiating reading groups about specific topics of interest to parents. The clergy are also moving out of traditional roles and having parent workshops regularly scheduled into the life of their churches and synagogues.

Parents independently are getting into the act as well. Recently, I was called in by an activist mother who was organizing a group of sixth-grade parents to establish a set of common guidelines regarding their kids' burgeoning social lives. It included a "safe house" contract, signed by each parent, attesting that an adult would always be present when adolescent friends got together in their homes, that no child would ever leave alone, and that no alcohol would be served or drugs tolerated. Enough parents agreed to the contract to form the nucleus of a parent community that could share information of common concern about their children. The very fact that each parent or set of parents knew that the guidelines they supported would be backed up by other families gave them a sense of strength in numbers that reinforced their own authority.

This is an example of how parents can strengthen each other. There are many other steps helping professionals can take to challenge the second family. Among them the following:

1. Encourage communication between parents. Without some compensating network of their own, parents are usually defeated by the barrier that frequently exists between them and their kids, kept rigidly in place by a strict code of silence enforced by the adolescent network. Violators of the code suffer the worst torment imaginable in the adolescent idea of hell: ostracism from the pack.

With the threat of exile hanging over their kids, parents often feel that they are held hostage to the peer group, unable to report to other parents something they have learned about a child's friend—that she is anorexic, using drugs, drinking, etc. The "phone tree" is another community-wide intervention we can support. Phone trees consist of the names of a group of parents who all have one another's numbers (their work numbers, if possible, so kids are less likely to hear "incriminating" telephone conversations). This provides a kind of witness protection program, with reasonable assurance of anonymity for parental tipsters.

When kids first hear about these plans, they are often furious: "What right do parents have to find out what is going on in our lives and monitor our whereabouts," demanded a group of 14- and 15-year-olds in a Midwestern Quaker school. To which the parents, strengthened in resolve by their new solidarity, could say without anger or defiance: "It's our job to protect and take care of our children; we'll do whatever is necessary."

When parents communicate, the kids can less easily play the adults off against each other or finger anyone as the informer. For example, Alice, the mother of a 14-year-old girl, found out about a party without supervision. She immediately activated the phone tree and, within a few hours, just about all the parents in the grade knew about it in time to discourage or direct their own kids not to go. Family therapists have long been right on this—no matter how energetic their initial resistance, kids are often deeply relieved when parents regain their authority. In fact, most adolescents will want their mothers and fathers to be part of the network. Diane, the mother of a 13-year-old, told me that, after I encouraged her to begin a parents group, one of her son's skinhead friends swaggered menacingly into her kitchen in full regalia—boots, chains, tattoos—and demanded to know why his Mom hadn't been invited to the group. "Next time, don't leave her out!" he ordered, before stomping out of the kitchen. Kids, even those in chains, feel better when we help create a neighborhood of parents—a "there" to hold and protect them.

2. Teach parents how to talk to the peer group. Professionals must help parents get to a teenager's friends and peers if they want to have any insight about the pressures, values, ideas, desires, fads, and events that define what is important to their child. But how do you do this apparently impossible task, when all kids seem intent on creating a permanent safe space between them and their hopelessly out-of-it parents? When fathers and mothers directly ask their own kid about the peer group, they are making a child feel torn between loyalties to both the primary and secondary families. But there are other, more direct ways to get to know what's going on.

Jesse, for example, a 15-year-old sophomore, had been inviting about a half-dozen friends over to his house on weekend nights. They regularly hung out together until 2 or 3 A.M. Despite incriminating evidence in the garage—cigarette packs, the odor of old pot and tobacco—his parents, Katherine and George, avoided doing anything until a small fire in the garage triggered a call to me. Holding Jesse accountable for his friends' actions was hopeless. I felt stymied and finally suggested that they talk directly to the second family kids themselves.

Katherine, George, and I rehearsed what they would say—no moralizing sermons, no outrage—just an expression of their feelings and consequences, much as I describe in Chapter 6. The next time Jesse and his friends met, the parents said, "We are not here because we want to make you do something 'for your own good,' or to 'build character,' or to 'show you who's boss,' but because we are so worried ourselves that we can't sleep. We are terrified that there will be a fire, that you might be injured or even killed, or just that somebody might drink too much, or smoke too much pot and be unable to get home safely. These are risks we cannot have." If Mom and Dad found, on weekly inspection, that the behavior continued, the garage would immediately be locked up. Because the message was delivered with dead seriousness and without appeals to morality, the kids did not protest. In fact, months later, Jesse admitted that he had been enormously relieved—the garage/night club evenings had gotten out of hand. But he didn't know how to change things without being accused of wimpiness by his friends. In the meantime, Jesse's friends continued to come over, but because there was no particular reason to confine themselves to the garage any more, they began drifting into the living room and kitchen. Reminding them of the principles of parallel communication, I asked Jesse's parents to make a point of being available and unshockable by the details of the kids' lives that had begun to emerge in the natural course of ordinary conversation. George and Katherine learned that one boy felt utterly rejected by his divorced mother, whom he never saw because she worked such long hours, that another had been beaten by his abusive father, and that a third suffered from severe learning difficulties, making his school life a living hell.

Over the course of a year and a half (no sudden transformation here), Katherine and George slowly began to make contact with the other parents, talking about their common problems, mentioning that they themselves were getting some counseling for the family "just to get us through Jesse's adolescence." One by one, each in their own way, the other families followed suit. At the 18-month anniversary of the original garage discussion, most of the kids, either with families or alone, had entered some program or counseling.

3. Strengthen the connection between parents and school. With the adult infrastructure so fragmented, today's mental health professionals can't rest until parents are talking to the schools where children spend the lion's share of their waking lives. Teachers and parents are often still as isolated as other neighborhood adults and inclined to mutual suspicion. Many teachers feel overworked and unappreciated; they complain that parents are too busy to spend time monitoring kids and then blame them (the teachers) for the D's and F's. Parents regularly complain that teachers are either too strict or too lenient, don't really try to know the children individually, or rarely understand their particular difficulties. This shifting of blame between home and school is yet another symptom of the already fragile nature of adult authority in kids' lives and another glaring reason counselors must move from working only with the family at home to reorganizing neighborhood systems.

A classic problem at school is the child who is taunted, and even physically harassed, by schoolmates. School authorities often do nothing and parents either feel too cowed by the school bureaucracy to complain or ignored by teachers when they do. Many parents (and counselors) try to deal with the problem at home, advising their child to "ignore the other kids." The road less traveled is that we must help parents and schools deal with the problem as a coordinated team.

Twelve-year-old Jason had just moved into a new school district and, being insecure, tried in all the wrong ways to get himself noticed and make friends. Unfortunately, Jason was noticed, but by the tough school bullies. These boys made Jason's life a torment—taunting him nastily every day, threatening him, and on several occasions roughing him up during breaks. Over the course of several months, Jason lost all interest in schoolwork, began having nightmares, and moped around the house, lonely and friendless.

Just working with the parents' dynamics had little impact on Jason's situation. Finally I suggested what should have been at the top of my agenda, that we create an alliance with the school. Approached directly, being asked to assist, not criticized or blamed, Jason's school responded quickly and effectively. The principal called every tormentor in, one by one, and said, "You don't have to like Jason or even talk to him. But you may not in any way insult, harass, or attack him. Anyone doing so will be suspended from school."

The other boys were initially furious at Jason for getting them in trouble, but because there was nothing to do about it, they left him alone. Just having some peace was such a relief to Jason that, within a month or two, he settled down and began doing his schoolwork. One day, Jason got on the school bus and, finding no other seats available, had to sit next to one of the less central members of the gang. During the course of the ride, the two began hesitantly to talk and discovered a common interest in computers. The exchange turned into a tentative friendship. Jason's mother encouraged him to have the boy over to their house and, eventually, a second and third classmate began turning up as well. Jason now has a small circle of friends—some of them his former enemies—with whom he eats lunch, plays, and enjoys a normal, happy social life.

Another example of how to act as facilitator or liaison between teachers and parents: Lauren, a 13-year-old eighth grader with an unaddressed reading disorder, attended school only about half the time, and, no matter what Margie, her mother, did or said, she could not get her daughter to attend regularly. Margie, in desperation, was taking her child to school daily, hanging around outside for an hour or so to make sure she stayed; but, not only did this put her own job in jeopardy, it proved useless since Lauren regularly skipped out anyway as soon as Margie left the scene. Parent and school were, once again, like estranged marriage partners, blaming each other for this scenario.

I spoke to Margie, the principal, and Lauren's teacher, telling them to put aside their mutual distrust and pointing out that it would hardly help the girl's academic life, not to mention her psychological state, to ignore the problem. With responsibility being equally divided and with Margie not viewed as an adversary, the principal applied herself to the problem with energy and imagination: "What if we let Lauren know that it is as important to us as to her mother that she go to school?" The principal then astonished me by giving Lauren a wake-up call: "Get yourself out of bed," she told Lauren, "and out the door to school where I will meet you and your mom. If you don't come, I will come and walk with both of you," the principal promised serenely.

Lauren felt so stunned by the knowledge that both her mother and the school were watching over her that she showed up and stayed the first day. We could now create a more coordinated effort to help Lauren, Mom, and school work together on her reading disorder. Six months later she is struggling to keep up with homework assignments (which are monitored weekly by a teacher–parent checklist) and has missed virtually no school.

4. Establish anonymous hot lines in schools. Looking for other structured ways to create cohesion between disconnected parts of the adolescent context, I have since encouraged schools to establish a confidential hot line that allows kids to anonymously get help for friends in trouble. Even as I lobbied school administrations to become involved, I privately wondered whether secretive teens would make use of the service. I was, in fact, surprised—kids immediately began calling. Recently, for example, one nameless 14-year-old girl called the hot line to report the severe bulimia of a friend, Beth (who, obviously realizing she was in trouble, had told several buddies about her binging, vomiting, and laxative cycle). The counselor called Beth in and said that "A lot of your friends are very worried about you, and we are, too." Because Beth was hesitant about speaking, and obviously afraid of telling her parents, the counselor asked her if it would be easier to talk with her best friend, Lenore, present. After a few meetings with the two girls—discussing the social pressures to be thin, the feeling of self-hatred if they gained weight—Beth felt confident enough to give the counselor permission to call her parents. Her mom and dad were enormously relieved—they had suspected problems but did not really know how to approach their increasingly distant child.

Eventually, as Beth and her family began to deal with the bulimia, the school, with Beth contributing behind the scenes, initiated an educational program about eating disorders, involving kids, teachers, and parents. It included films and presentations by experts in the area. As a result of the program, several other girls in the same grade went to the counselor admitting to their eating disorders. What had been the terrible problem of one isolated teenager, shrouding her second family of peers in deepest secrecy, had become a shared community issue.

5. Create peer groups for parents. Given that one of the major problems today is a lack of connection between the adults in a child's life, one of the most powerful interventions is to get parent groups started. Whether you're a teacher, counselor, or school administrator, anyone who works directly with teens can understand the value in promoting better communication in the adult network. Almost every example I've given in this chapter could have been less serious if parents had been talking to each other all along. The major considerations necessary to form such a group are listed in the accompanying box.

＊　　　＊　　　＊

Peer Groups for Parents

Groups of parents can truly strengthen the authority and compassion of adults in a community. Follow these steps to create one in your area:

1. Begin a group when there's motivation—usually this is after a crisis.
2. Make sure the school administration is on board.
3. Include parents of kids in the same grade.
4. Find two energetic parents to organize the group.
5. Meet as often as parents can handle—once a month or every other month is usually workable.
6. Ask parents to sign a confidentiality agreement—so rumors don't spread.
7. Lead the group until the process is established.
8. Train parents as group facilitators.
9. The content of group meetings can be readings, guest speakers, or discussions about everyday life.
10. Remember, the group is used to increase communication—not to legislate rules for the kids.

Creating this synergism is not glamorous, but more a matter of stitching together the different parts in the life of a troubled teen. This is what many of us have been privately doing all along. But it doesn't happen easily; on the contrary, I know I'm doing the job right just when it feels as if I am on the edge of failure, just when I think I can't take it anymore. The work is so demanding I've come to the conclusion that none of us should, or even can, handle a practice entirely devoted to adolescents.

The bottom line is that the adult world, so isolated from the world of adolescents, so frenetic in its pace, needs to become more connected in order to deal with the current crisis. If we adults don't take these steps to create our own functioning adult network, our children will most certainly fall through the cracks.

chapter eight

Resilient Kids

Nurturing Self-Esteem in 21st-Century
Children and Adolescents

After working with kids for 25 years, it is clear
to me that there are few issues more critical
than their self-esteem. Unfortunately, our mental health and teaching fields have contributed to some of the self-esteem difficulties of today's children—not by negligence or less than worthy intentions, but by a rigid mind-set about building self-esteem. The belief that one should feel special "just for being" has proven far from successful. New research on resilience has demonstrated what works and what doesn't in strengthening kids' confidence. And, as professionals on the front lines, we should be aware of the latest findings about how to create greater resilience in our young clients.

The Hidden Signals of Low Self-Esteem

Today, kids present quite differently than just one or two decades ago. Most children don't come in with overt symptoms of inadequacy that blatantly signal self-esteem deficits. Usually they present with much more confidence and only upon closer examination reveal the *hidden* signs of low self-esteem. Because red flag indicators are changing for this core attribute, we professionals need to know the half-dozen signals that a child, no matter how outwardly sturdy, needs help to restore her self-esteem.

Few Adult Mentors in a Child's Life

Research shows that among the biggest influences on development are teachers, coaches, or spiritual group leaders—in other words, responsible adults. Yet, as I have discussed in Chapter 7, in modern culture the adult and child worlds run in parallel universes, so these relationships are surprisingly difficult to come by. Child-centered activities, TV programs, indeed, entire TV stations devoted to kids—MTV, VH1, Nickelodeon—make it all too easy for youngsters to become disconnected from real-life adults. The gradual alienation between the generations begins not during adolescence, as it did decades ago, but for more vulnerable kids as early as first and second grades. In addition, today's children are scheduled into so many different activities that only a few remain involved with adult mentors long term. By the time adolescence hits, kids rarely hang out with grown-ups outside their families and, as the chance for adult guidance decreases, the chance for risky behavior skyrockets.

A Fund of Basic Information, yet a Profound Disinterest in Reading

Most children I meet read few books for their own enjoyment. I am constantly surprised by how little interest there is in the written word, especially compared to pop culture pursuits—TV, movies, the Internet, and video games. For many 21st century kids, books are typically thought of as tie-ins to movies or TV shows. Standardized testing has documented my clinical observations—lower reading proficiency scores, little or no knowledge of history, the increasing failure of schools to meet newly established state guidelines, etc. Most of the troubled kids I meet have long before given up on reading; instead, they derive most of their knowledge from the pop culture.

For example, Jacob, was a boy I met when he was 11 years old and who got into a mess of trouble in school—failing classes, not wanting to do homework, and being increasingly defiant to the adults in his life. Despite his failing grades, Jacob was surprisingly conversant about all current events and contemporary issues. He was a veritable compendium of "factoids" and spoke in the most animated way. As I got past Jacob's facade, it became quite clear that all his information had been gleaned from the pop culture, TV headlines between his favorite sitcoms, sound bites from talk shows, and overheard conversations. In fact, Jacob had not read a single book since first grade.

Without basic comfort in the written word, many challenging pursuits become difficult, if not impossible. This leads to a miles-wide but inch-deep attitude vis-à-vis learning, a stance that has a direct impact on a child's inner sense of competence. Much of the swagger, trash talk, and rudeness I've witnessed hides a disregard, even contempt, for the demanding nature of activity that requires work to gain mastery.

A Child Is Glib, yet Has Difficulty Actually Saying Anything about What Truly Matters

Many millennium kids are proficient at what I call "popspeak." They come in under the worst circumstances: about to be expelled from school, in deep trouble with their families, perhaps having a history of substance abuse. Despite these negative circumstances, they can be very verbal and surprisingly cordial. Yet, after we talk, I realize that I haven't learned anything about what is going on inside them. Here's an example of popspeak. The following dialogue occurred when I met with 12-year-old Anna:

DR. T: So, what do you think about what just happened between your mom and you?

ANNA: It's all right. [They'd just had an enormous argument over schoolwork.]

DR. T: All right?

ANNA: Yeah. Yeah.

DR. T: Well, what did you *feel* about the fight between you and your mom? Were you angry? Were you sad?

ANNA: Not really, well, maybe a little. Yeah. You know what? I can relate to my mom. She was just sort of like in a bad frame. She's like . . . like, wow, "I'm a mom and that's what I'm supposed to do." You know what I mean?

DR. T: Sort of.

ANNA: Well. You know how Sabrina's [a TV character] aunts are? She's a little like that, a little "much." I mean, if I were a witch I definitely would be wearing different clothes. Let's face it. She's like "Oh, my God, look how dressy I can get for school!" . . . Do you get what I'm saying?

This glib noncommunication is typical for children with low self-esteem and has been described by school consultant Michael Nerney as lack of "emotional literacy." The inability to express the emotions that really matter damages a child's self-esteem for the following reasons:

1. It is hard to ask for advice without being able to express oneself.
2. Disturbing feelings remain internalized and either create symptoms or anger.
3. It is difficult to translate troublesome emotions into constructive action.
4. Connections and alliances are made with other nonverbal kids.
5. Without responsible adult guidance, risky behaviors are more likely.

A Child Has Interests, but Mostly in Nonhierarchical Pursuits

Many traditional hobbies have rules of engagement, steps toward mastery, and clear guidelines for how one progresses from point A to point B. Just think of chess, ballet, or even stamp collecting. This old-fashioned notion of "practice" is being replaced by activities in which kids can do well without rules imposed by adults; instead, whatever rules exist are child created and controlled (e.g., Nintendo or computer games). These do nothing to solidify a child's tolerance for frustration, nor do they add to a sense of authentic competence. Over time, the inability to do much without immediate payback becomes a major source of low self-esteem.

For example, 14-year-old Julia had a vivid way of describing this problem. "Ron," she said quite candidly, "I've been playing computer games for as long as I can remember. I'm used to getting an immediate reward. When I think about doing schoolwork or continuing in gymnastics like my parents want me to, all I can think about is that it's not 'so fun.' I guess I'm saying the hard work doesn't seem worth it. I didn't like having to drop out of the gym class but so what, in the end who really cares?"

Learning Problems Are Kept at Arms' Length

Some children make it extremely difficult for a parent to find out what's really going on in the world of schoolwork. Many kids actively shield this realm from adult eyes; they won't let them see homework or get involved with academic projects. This is a red flag that self-esteem about accomplishment is overshadowed by shame about the inability to learn.

For example, James had been identified as being extremely bright as early as preschool. He even was accepted into a program for gifted children. Kindergarten with its emphasis on play and group projects was a breeze for James. First grade, however, became somewhat more difficult. The teacher assigned monthly homework projects, and James always put up a fuss before settling down to complete them. As demands became greater in second and third grade, James adopted a kind of smart-ass attitude towards his parents and even his teachers. He projected an image of a kid who was more interested in the pop culture than being in school. Fundamental to his ability to get by was James's increasing skill at keeping his schoolwork cordoned off from his parents. James's excuse-making talents became almost legendary: "I left the assignment in my locker"; "Oh, I just remembered that it's due tomorrow"; "Don't look my homework over—I want it to be mine." Finally, the teachers and his parents had a conference and recognized just how uncomfortable James was with his basic academic skills. He was so smart he could conceal his difficulty comprehending multisyllabic words, complex thoughts, and paragraphs. Sadly, this conference occurred in third grade, 2 years after he'd begun hiding out from the important adults around. Had they picked up on the not-so-subtle signals, remediation would have begun earlier.

Difficulty Absorbing Praise about Accomplishments

Some kids have a terrible time accepting compliments. Parents, teachers, and counselors report that it's hard to praise—children downplay or look away even as positive feedback is offered. It is almost as if positive feedback doesn't feel consistent with the authentic self. This is another red flag that a child's self-esteem needs attention. For example, Darren, a 12-year-old boy with an undiagnosed learning problem, feels fraudulent. Like many such children, Darren had created a false-self identity with adults. Smiling, seemingly compliant, he spent his grade-school years developing masterful ways of "just getting by." The adults, impressed with his obvious intelligence, had high hopes for him: they did not see, as Darren harshly put it, his real identity—a "lazy, lying, slacker" whose major pursuit was "outsmarting all the grown-ups around." For years, teachers and parents mistakenly believed that positive stroking was going to make a difference. But Darren knew how much he didn't know. Instead of feeling better, he actually became more sullen and contemptuous when complimented. Finally, a teacher broke through by recognizing Darren's learning difficulties, addressing for the first time what the boy really needed—remediation, not praise.

Popularity Rules

For many kids with self-esteem problems, popularity becomes *the* most important aspect of life, usually hiding some inadequacy in

learning and school performance. Today, this obsession is mass produced by the pop culture and preoccupies vulnerable children at
earlier and earlier ages, even in kindergarten and first grade. By first
grade many boys and girls already wear the latest designer labels,
make fun of "nerdier" kids, are completely fluent in popspeak and
trends. Over the years, especially if learning issues persist, popularity takes over as the prime drive toward mastery. A child's resilience
is truly at risk because, lacking an inner sense of confidence or competence, she depends on belonging, fitting into the cooler groups,
and on the admiring reactions from other kids.

For example, a wonderful girl named Cindy whom I met when
she was a sixth grader described to me her own struggles with
"popularity." Cindy was an extremely bright, highly articulate, but
not stunningly gorgeous kid. She wasn't rich, nor did she dress in a
"cool" way. But, most important, she lacked one of the key compo-
nents of popularity. Cindy: "I want to be with the popular girls,
and sometimes I think about it so much I don't feel like doing my
schoolwork. But all the popular kids seem to like to put each other
down. I don't want to have to do that to be accepted—but, at the
same time, I want to be accepted more than anything else. What
should I do?"

Popularity is really about the authentic self not being good
enough without continuous admiration from peers and without
feeling superior to those around.

Why Self-Esteem Is Increasingly at Risk in Today's Children

To further recognize the subtle signals of low self-esteem, it helps
to understand some of the social/political forces that fuel the current assault on kids' resilience. This increases the possibility of spotting troubled children early on—in the classroom, guidance office,
or activity groups—and informs advice to parents. Because the
forces that chip away at core self-worth are endemic to society, recognizing them also creates greater empathy toward parents, who
are never solely responsible for a child's difficulties in the self-
esteem area.

Until the Mid-to-Late 1990s, We Have Been Expecting Less from Our Kids

In the last few years, there are some positive signs: for example, girls' math SAT scores have been rising, but the general news on achievement scores has not been positive. Many children feel—and in my opinion this is a consequence of the self-esteem movement—*it's enough if they just show up*. Twenty-five years ago, some states even made self-esteem a "right," which legitimized a sense of entitlement without proving competence:

- As reported by Charles J. Sykes in *Dumbing Down Our Kids* (St. Martin's Press, 1996), testing reveals that we are one of the lower-rated industrial nations in terms of reading and math achievement. In addition, knowledge of fundamental history and geography facts has slowly been declining.
- Grade inflation, as reported in *U.S. News and World Report* ("Best Colleges—Annual Guide," June, 1999), has eroded nearly 15% off a child's true grade—schools wanting to show better college placement award higher grades for lower performance.
- According to the College Board, the proportion of students taking SATs with an A average rose from 28% to 37% from 1987 to 1997, even though combined test scores *fell* 14 points.
- As states recognized widespread academic weakness and proposed new and tougher standards, they have become overwhelmed by the numbers of kids who can't conform to the new guidelines.
- Parents repeatedly report that awards for younger children in schools, extracurricular activities, and skill groups are increasingly for participation rather than merit.

As these examples indicate, kids are encouraged to feel self-esteem regardless of how well they perform. Psychologist Mary Pipher pointedly asks, "Do we want to make children feel good about themselves, rather than actually *being* good?" Many educators agree with Pipher. For example, in an article that appeared on *The New York Times* op-ed page (July 15, 1993), Lillian Katz, a professor of early childhood education, cites a bulletin board in one school hallway entitled, "We Applaud Ourselves." As Katz points out, "The poster urged self-congratulation; yet it made no reference to possible ways of *earning* applause." She also comments on a kindergarten classroom in which children completed the sentence "I am special because . . . " with phrases such as "I can color," "I can ride a bike," and "I like to play with my friends." Making a child feel "special" for such common, average accomplishments, says Katz, is destined to rebound: "If everybody is special, nobody is special."

Entitlement Is Fueled by the Second Family's Consumerism

Materialism saps a child's sense of intrinsic self-worth. The pop culture encourages kids to be on the lookout for more. Children feel they're not good enough unless they have "the right stuff." No matter what socioeconomic class they belong to, kids need the gear.

For example, 8-year-old Alex wants to be one step ahead of all his friends. Specifically, Alex is into what Mel Levine calls "future-wanting" (*Educational Care*, Educator's Publishing Service, 1994). This means that Alex is highly tuned into the movies, the product tie-ins, and the latest action figures that are just about to be released. He never seems happy with what he has in the present. As soon as he sees a new toy or exciting gear being advertised, he needs to have it as well. The problem is that constantly needing *more* makes a child feel *empty* inside. You never are enough unless you have enough.

The Culture of Speed

An article by James Gleik in *The New York Times* entitled "Addicted to Speed" (*New York Times Magazine*, September 28, 1997) described that we are programmed to think so quickly, we are "hooked" on action. The average child and adult changes channels 20 times a minute. The average length of time for a TV scene is down from 30 seconds to cuts that last no more than 1 or 2 seconds. TV producers are so afraid of our twitchy remote control habits, they've even done away with credits at the end of shows—split screens highlight what's coming up next, just in case we get the urge to move on.

Of course, kids reflect our attitudes—and adults model frenetic behavior. We complain about kids needing instant gratification, yet our grown-up world is increasingly *built* on instant gratification. Computers, e-mail, technological wizardry—the list is endless—are all conceived with the idea that fast is good, but fastest is best.

Thus, pop psychology and everyday home life assaults kids with constant messages that undermine mastery and competence (see the accompanying box).

These messages disconnect children from authentic core self-experiences: passion, compassion, gratitude, pride in competency, motivation, expressiveness, and respect—experiences that are essential for true self-esteem.

Our job as professionals is to get kids reconnected to an authentic self even as the second family is pulling kids *away* from their personal center toward that which is external. Our task as teachers, counselors, and group leaders is to spot the hidden cues of self-esteem difficulties and help parents strengthen in children the kind of authentic self that promotes greater resilience.

What Builds Self-Esteem in Children

The research cited below describes recent trends in creating resilience, and would be extremely beneficial to share with your colleagues and with the families you meet. This growing body of evidence can add to your authority when you offer advice. Fortunately there is now persuasive research documenting what actually helps develop strong self-esteem.

Warmth Builds Self-Esteem

The latest studies by psychologist Jerome Kagan indicate that the earliest roots of self-esteem come from primary parent–child inter-

Trying Is for Nerds

Adults aren't always aware of how the deck is stacked against pride in mastery. Here are just a few of the anticompetency values that bombard kids from all directions:

1. You're special because you're *you*.
2. Expect praise simply for *participating*.
3. Don't think—*just do it*.
4. Yesterday doesn't count. Today is old. *Tomorrow has what you want*.
5. Smart is *geeky*.
6. Passion is for *nerds*.
7. *More* is better.
8. Do it *faster*.
9. You're *not enough* unless you *have* enough.
10. *Get the stuff!*.

actions. Warmth and accurate empathic responses impact on brain structure and shape it differently than does a less affectionate environment. In child developmentalist Stanley I. Greenspan's words, "Nurture affects nature" (*The Growth of the Mind*, Addison-Wesley, 1997). Not that parents and professionals didn't intuitively know this. But now contemporary researchers are able to show that interpersonal warmth actually changes neural patterning in the brain. Successful early bonding is associated with later ability to learn concepts, greater curiosity, and emotional intelligence. All of these traits, of course, are building blocks for a sense of resilience.

If the kids you meet weren't fortunate enough to have had such warmth and acceptance early on, don't give up. Researchers Alan Sroufe and June Fleeson of the University of Minnesota have done almost a hundred studies of parent–child attachment and have concluded that through adolescence, children's personalities are very plastic—loving relationships with adults, even in later stages of development, still change interpersonal patterns for the better.

Storytelling Builds Self-Esteem

Jerome Bruner is another researcher redefining our view of self-esteem. One of his major contributions is the importance of "storytelling" between parent and child (*Acts of Meaning*, Harvard University Press, 1990). The act of storytelling, a time-worn child-rearing practice, has also been proven to positively affect brain structure *and* to further a powerful connection between parent and child. These, in turn, strengthen resilience. Spoken stories, even for kids who are infants and unable to understand them, are important. This is because the soothing cadence and tone of the narrative help a child connect with his caregiver in a way that builds a secure sense of self—one of the foundations of genuine self-esteem. It communicates the protective messages "You are safe," "You are accepted," "You are loved."

Emotional Literacy Builds Self-Esteem

A third foundation of self-esteem is suggested by the work of communication expert Michael Nerney. As described above, most kids with low self-esteem don't have what he calls "emotional literacy." These children can't put their feelings into words. Instead, they act out in ways that are unreflective and ultimately self-destructive. Problems with expressiveness are obvious in the classroom or by the time kids are seen by helping professionals. Teachers and counselors work with children to help them identify feelings and take constructive actions to resolve them. In these ways we help kids develop the expressiveness that is associated with what psychologist Dan Stern calls "personal agency": I know what I feel. I express myself effectively enough to be taken care of and to take care of myself (*The Interpersonal World of the Infant*, Basic Books, 1985).

Proper Praise Builds Self-Esteem

The fourth area undergoing a significant change is in the realm of learning theory—what kind of praise helps kids *learn* to feel greater self-esteem. Edward Deci, author of *Why We Do What We Do*

(Putnam, 1995), proposes the following counterintuitive idea: the *more* we praise and reward children for learning, the *less* they want to learn. The true reward of doing a task, the research indicates, is *doing the task!* Performance doesn't have to be a success, or even lauded as one. It is the effort and completion of the task that matter. Therefore, when we reward kids regularly, they lose interest in the job. Helping parents understand when and how to praise kids is a powerful tool in building perseverance. And perseverance, the ability to stick with frustration, is a necessary component of solid self-esteem.

Optimism Builds Self-Esteem

The fifth foundation of self-esteem currently being redefined is described in work done by Martin E. P. Seligman, author of *The Optimistic Child* (Houghton Mifflin, 1995), Seligman presents research spanning 20 years which shows that kids do not do well receiving *excessive praise,* for example, when well-meaning teachers and parents say they're the *"absolute best"* or that they've just done the *"most amazing* job ever!" Hyperbolic praise causes children to think of themselves as fraudulent. Seligman's work is a powerful critique of the parenting literature and particularly of the self-esteem movement. What cognitive researchers suggest may sound hurtful to many modern professionals schooled in unending praise: *Honest, realistic feedback is what builds self-esteem.* Seligman's "realistic feedback" is a phrase that can sound harsh to self-esteem-obsessed adults. However, everyday experience with kids shows that realistic feedback, kindly delivered, *does* lead to more accurate and compassionate self-appraisal. And an accurate view of oneself makes it more possible to take constructive action and find eventual satisfaction in mastery (see the accompanying box).

"Constructive Criticism" Diminishes Self-Esteem

The contributions of parenting experts originally trained by Alice and Haim Ginott, authors of *Between Parent and Child* (Morrow/ Avon, 1967)—namely, Adele Faber and Elaine Mazlich, authors of

---

"Kindness" That Kills Motivation versus Realistic Feedback That Inspires

Parents and professionals often associate realistic feedback with being unempathic or destructive. The difference is great and ought to be understood by all adults trying to get through to children. Here are some examples:

INAPPROPRIATE PRAISE	REALISTIC FEEDBACK
"That was great!"	"You've done better in the past."
"You're the best in the group."	"You're one of the better readers in your group."
"That was terrific—you tried your best."	"It's true, you didn't really put in your best effort."

How to Talk So Kids Will Listen (Morrow/Avon, 1999); Nancy Samalin, *Loving Your Child Is Not Enough* (Viking Penguin, 1987); and Lawrence Balter, *Who's In Control* (Simon & Schuster, 1988)—are wonderful resources that show the damage of constructive criticism. These authors suggest alternatives that I will describe later in this chapter. How can constructive criticism (which many of us grew up with) be bad for self-esteem? Experience has taught us that when parents "constructively criticize," kids do not hear the constructive intention, they usually hear the criticism. Lessening this negativity between parent and child can be a powerful tool toward building genuine self-esteem (see the accompanying box).

How to Nurture Self-Esteem

Recent trends in the research I've described above lead to a better understanding of how resilience in modern children is continuously undermined and inform several key strategies to work on with par-

Criticism: Destructive versus Constructive

Many of us were brought up by parents and teachers who used supposedly constructive criticism to improve or to correct unwanted behaviors. Unfortunately, the effect is not always one that produces the desired results. Nor does it build confidence or motivation. Here are some ways to subtly turn unwittingly hurtful comments into corrective statements that build resilience in kids.

DESTRUCTIVE	CONSTRUCTIVE
"You're too stubborn for your own good."	"Sometimes you act in a stubborn way."
"A 90 percent is good but what happened to those other 10 points?"	"That was terrific . . . and I know you could do even better."
"You need to stop leaving everything on the floor. You're a slob, exactly like your father."	"Some of your behaviors, like not picking up after yourself, remind me of your father."

ents. Keep these strategies in mind when dealing with any parent or child in which you spot the hidden signals of low self-esteem:

1. Lessen parental criticism. Guide mothers and fathers to help kids develop greater resilience by lessening the amount of criticism at home. First, since criticism is often out of awareness, ask parents to keep a log of interactions. As described in Chapter 1, parents need only jot down a couple of scenarios. Another more dramatic technique that uncovers subtle criticism is for a parent to leave a tape recorder in the dining room, or perhaps on the kitchen table where the family gathers. After a few days the recorder disappears in the rubble of daily living and no one notices it. The parent can later listen to everyday dialogues. Suddenly, in the starkest fashion possible, he or she hears the damaging messages that have been taken for granted. Here are some common but subtle criticisms that parents discover after writing stories from home or listening to actual tape recordings:

   a. Comparisons. One type of criticism is extremely widespread—comparing your child to yourself, other people, a sibling, or a friend (see the accompanying box).

   b. Assuming. "I know what you're feeling"; "I've felt the same thing myself"; "I understand exactly." These phrases seem innocuous enough, even comforting. But if we repeatedly assume we know what our kids mean, we're often wrong. (I've learned this talking with kids every day for decades.) For example, a parent recently told me this amusing story: 5- or 6-year old Becky was sitting in the car, and the Clinton affair was being discussed on the radio. All of a sudden Becky said, "Mom, Dad, what does it mean to be 'brought up on charges for oral sex'?" The parents of this youngster were, of course, stunned. They immediately launched into a detailed, hesitant and very nervous explanation: "Oh my God . . . well, oral sex, well . . . " And Becky said, "No, no—what does it mean to be *brought up on charges?*"

   Assuming of this sort becomes even more of a problem with an older child. Twelve-year-old Jamie, speaking for many kids her age, said, "I can't stand it when my parents try to read my mind. They think they know exactly what I mean—when they haven't got a

---

Comparisons Hurt

Everyone compares. It's human nature and impossible to entirely eradicate. But interviews with kids have shown that particular comparisons are especially destructive. Help parents work on criticisms—

- Made in a moment of rage
- Made in front of siblings or friends
- Made as a blanket statement about character
- Made when a child already feels bad about an event
- That are justified, but said in a disparaging tone
- That are laced with subtle but noticeable sarcasm

clue." The stakes of this miscommunication are particularly danger-ous. Out of resentment and frustration, teens like Jamie clam up entirely and develop a negative mind-set about communicating with their parents that can last well into young adulthood.

Every day as a therapist I learn the same painful lesson: if I as-sume that I know what they're thinking, I rarely understand what kids are trying to tell me. So, help parents not think they "always know." Chronic errors in empathy make children think their feel-ings are *incorrect* and their true self is not being heard.

c. Pushing for "just one more." One of the more subtle criticisms a parent can make of a child is when he or she is unsatis-fied with what a child does—and asks for "just one more." Most parents can relate to this phenomenon as it occurs around meal-times. A child finishes his plate, and Mom or Dad, with the best in-tentions, pushes for him to take "one more bite." It seems so harm-less, perhaps even helpful, but in fact, over time, these kinds of exchanges communicate the idea: "You don't know your own appe-tites or needs—*I* do!" As children become older, the struggle over "getting it right" moves into many other activities: fashion, hand-writing, schoolwork, choice of friends, etc. In each of these areas, many well-meaning parents will find just a tiny little something to comment on: "Maybe this blouse would look nicer if . . . "; "You forgot to dot that 'i' . . . "; "Try one more math problem . . . "; and so on.

This subtle form of criticism can become part of the very fabric of the parent–child relationship. In almost every such situation I've encountered, the child develops a nagging sense of self-doubt.

2. Demand an ongoing interest. Help mothers and fathers encourage a substantial sense of self in children by demanding an ongoing interest. One passion in addition to schoolwork is essen-tial. Pop culture, with it's emphasis on consumerism and superficial knowledge is not a sufficient area of interest. I define a constructive interest as something that—

a. **is participatory,**
b. **has rules,**
c. **is a skill that improves with practice,**

d. demands a level of growing competence, and
e. includes adult mentors.

Such constructive interest can be as varied as soccer or stamp collecting. It is not always easy for parents to appreciate that one extracurricular activity can have a major impact. I describe how important this can be in Chapter 11.

Interests are particularly critical during the transition from elementary to middle school. Research shows a marked drop in kids' interests between sixth and seventh grade, a change that profoundly affects self-esteem. The Johnson Institute in Minnesota has followed thousands of children over several decades. The researchers found that kids were less prone toward substance abuse and other self-destructive behaviors if, during this transitional time, they kept up self-care habits. Not surprisingly, without supervision every measure of self-care goes down: seventh graders dress more poorly, change their clothes less frequently, eat much less nutritionally, sleep and bathe less (The Johnson Institute/Student View Survey, *High Risk Transitions,* 1993).

If this measurable decline in self-care *is accompanied by withdrawing from pursuits or interests*, the stage is set for potential acting out. Every month I meet teens who were once soccer freaks, baseball card afficionados, or into art. Sadly, they lose interest between sixth and eighth grades and begin hanging out with more marginal groups in school—those vulnerable to risky behaviors. Tell parents to fight this developmental vulnerability. When an ongoing interest is expected of children, parents are implicitly saying, "I want to try to protect your true self." This is an important message against the power of the second family—the huge network of peers and pop culture that by middle school communicates the message that being really good at something is not "cool." Because of the second family's strength, we need to help parents give kids the courage to be able to do things that are not cool. Protecting self-esteem doesn't stop with just "saying no" to temptation. It's also about developing an interest—something that is a growing part of a child's core self.

3. Nurture a child's obsessions. A related strategy for promoting greater self-esteem is nurturing a child's obsessions. Obsessions are the fuel that ignites mastery. This is because an obsession usually diminishes a child's need for instant gratification; it helps him learn to plan, follow complex instructions, and deal with frustration. Most obsessions end up having a ripple effect—strengthening a skill which, in turn, builds an authentic sense of self.

For example, Martin was "crazed" about dinosaurs, which he collected by the hundreds. Martin was not the most socially adept youngster, but despite his shyness built a substantial sense of self around his dinosaur obsession. He couldn't process language well, yet through this interest Martin began to talk and develop friendships with other dino-buddies. Adults in the museum (and other places with programs about dinosaurs) took an interest in Martin, mentoring him during the early years of his interest. By fourth grade Martin's skills originally nurtured around the dino-obsession came into play and helped him become more socially adept.

Another example: 6-year-old Keith's obsession was art, and then the movie *Titanic* came along. So what did he do? He branched out from simply watching the film to drawing many pictures of the Titanic, culminating in a Titanic model built from cardboard. The next thing he did was create a CD–ROM game, with rules and prizes. Then he and his parents wrote a letter to a toy company describing his ideas for the game. Keith constructed a diorama and brought it into class for "Show and Tell," sparking the formation of a club which created strong connections with other "Titanic nuts" in the class. With the encouragement of Keith's teacher, Mom and Dad nurtured this obsession, indeed helping it along the way. This interest affected almost every area of Keith's life, enabling him to move on to better relationships with kids in his class.

Praise That Gets Through to Children

Many parents don't know how to effectively praise children. We expect that expressions of pride are going to get through just because they're "positive." Parents often need to learn how to praise children in ways that truly build self-esteem. Based on the research cited above and specific vulnerabilities of 21st century children, here are the keys to praising children effectively; keep these in mind when counseling or guiding parents:

1. Praise when a child is ready to hear. Help parents see that children must be *ready* to accept praise. Just because adults are proud, that particular moment may not be when a child is able to absorb praise. Here's an example of when a child is *not* ready: Peter's just lost a game and feels badly about it. At that point, many well-meaning adults would try to give a pep talk about focusing on the bright side. This is precisely the *opposite* of what cognitive researchers like Martin Seligman suggest. In fact, the way to build strength is, as Peter's savvy coach did, to give realistic feedback: "You know, you're right, you *didn't* do as well today as on other days." It is extremely difficult to get most parents to say something negative; it feels almost mean. And yet, realistic feedback is exactly what helps a child's self-esteem grow.

The pull to offer unwarranted praise also happens in professional exchanges with kids who are upset. Teachers and counselors, for example, listen to what children are experiencing and then immediately try to get across a hopeful reframe, create motivation to take constructive action and encourage a mind-set that puts the event into perspective. But, no different with us than with their parents, kids don't hear our unwarranted praise either. Instead, we ought to offer realistic appraisals, kindly delivered. A wise teacher of my daughter had intuitively understood this when she said to Leah, "You're right. Getting the lead part in the play is a tremendous long shot. How do you think you'll feel if Ginny gets it?" Just as the research suggests, Leah heard this feedback, tried harder, and got a good supporting role—one she'd never had landed without her teacher's pointed but kindly words.

2. Avoid praising every time. As I've said, the self-esteem movement encourages parents to praise regularly and generously. Unfortunately, lavish stroking loses it's value and doesn't necessarily lead to greater resilience. For example, Claire is trying to offer praise because her daughter, Katelin, is dressing herself. She says with each step, "That's great. Good job. Good work!" Yet, at that moment, Katelin's auditory channel, her ability to hear this verbal praise, happens to be *off*. Not to be thwarted, Claire just keeps trying to get through, saying it even louder. But louder doesn't make it better. So, Claire ups the ante and becomes even more hyperbolic: "Wow. What a phenomenal job! You're the best." Still no reply.

A better strategy is to praise *once*. Tell parents that sometimes once *is* enough! If a child's not registering, save the good words for later. For example, after speaking with the guidance counselor, Claire adopted this approach: One morning when Katelin almost entirely dressed herself, Mom refrained from commenting and took her to school without mentioning a word about Katelin's improvement. Later that evening in a casual off-handed way, Claire briefly mentioned it: "The way you dressed yourself this morning sure seemed to start the day off better for both of us," and without waiting for a reply, continued cooking dinner for the family. Later that night, Claire overheard Katelin telling her dad proudly, "This morning, Daddy, I was really good. I got dressed all by myself!" Being attuned to when a child is open for praise avoids frustration and disconnection between parents and kids.

3. Don't make a big deal out of ordinary events. Again, parents have been encouraged to believe that every act of a child is "praiseworthy." For example, it had snowed heavily and the neighborhood kids were sleigh riding. Bringing my kids out to enjoy the snow, I found myself stunned by the frenetic self-esteem building going on all around me. As 3- and 4-year-olds slid merrily down the little hill, well-meaning parents furiously cheered them on: "Good job! Great work! Fantastic!" The kids, of course, didn't respond much, looking slightly perplexed by their parents' reactions. I couldn't help but think to myself, "What's happened to us? Now we have to praise children for 'accomplishing' something as natural as sleigh riding?"

This is a stark metaphor that tells volumes about how far afield we've come with the notion of praise. A good rule of thumb for modern parents is to praise the effort not the product. Praise determination, because how hard one tries is what feels genuine to kids (and adults). Good work ought to be commented on casually, with no fanfare, bells, or whistles.

4. Don't label the whole child. Adults should try to avoid saying: "You *are* a _____!" or "You *always* were _____." Help parents stay away from the following words: *everytime, never,* and *always*. These all-inclusive phrases make criticism hurtful rather than helpful. Instead, share criticism in the context of something that was positive about the effort—if you can do it genuinely. For example, Jenny just drew a picture in class. Truthfully, it was a half-hearted effort at best. Jenny's teacher, whom I'd spoken with earlier, said nothing. But, sometime later, after Jenny put real effort into another project, her teacher jumped on the opportunity, *praising the effort* and then referring back to her less spirited work: "You really tried much harder on this piece than the one before—and it shows!"

Criticism can be useful if it's realistic and doesn't negatively label the child's entire character.

Thinking Increases Self-Esteem

In thousands of pervasive ways, the pop culture pushes children to act without thinking. Because we professionals deal with acting-out kids every day, we must help parents teach children to think about the impact of their behaviors on themselves and others. To this end, I refer you to a wonderful book called *Raising a Thinking Child* by Myrna Shure (Holt, 1995). Using research with thousands of young children, Shure has developed an interpersonal-cognitive technique that helps a child identify his inner experience and then think about how his actions will make other people feel. Shure's strategies can be used with kids as young as 3 years old. Follow-up studies suggest that children trained in this technique are involved in fewer problem behaviors and an increased ability to problem-solve.

Simply put, the some of the more important steps are as follows:

- Help a child express experience in feeling terms. *Example*: "Did that fight with Suzanne make your feel glad, bad, or sad?"
- Practice with kids the ability to distinguish between "difference": before–after, good–bad, right–wrong, etc. This helps a child make distinctions between the effects of different behaviors. *Example*: "Was it right or wrong to make fun of Jamie?" or "Did you feel good or bad when you shared that toy?"
- Encourage kids to think ahead. "What do you think it will be like; how do you think it will make others feel?" *Example*: "How do you think Bobby will feel if you tell him that you don't want to sit next to him in school?" This encourages kids to reflect about the impact of their actions on other children.
- Ask problem-solving questions: "Can you think of another way to say it to Bobby so that he doesn't feel quite so bad?" Practicing solutions not only strengthens thinking but also creates greater flexibility in kids.

Each of these steps encourages a different aspect of reflection. Positive outcome reinforces the notion that thinking ahead feels good: A new friend is made. Classmates are nicer. A play date goes better. Because kids get satisfying feedback, motivation to think ahead again is created, further strengthening the positive experience of thinking ahead.

Looks Matter

Children's self-esteem is profoundly shaped by our culture's obsession with beauty. The forces of narcissism are insidious:

- According to a 1998 *New York Times*/CBS News poll of American teenagers, when they were asked the one thing they'd like to change about themselves, the most frequent answer from girls and boys alike was "My looks" or "My body."*

- In a Cincinnati study that surveyed *third-grade* boys and girls, 29% of the boys and 39% of the girls had already dieted.
- A California study determined that 81% of 10-year-old girls were or already had been on a diet.
- A national survey in the late 1980s showed that 90% of American girls *and* boys were unhappy with their weight.

Kids are reporting difficulties with body image and feeling inadequate at earlier ages than just a decade ago. Yet, despite these disturbing trends, relatively little has been written on how professionals can help parents fight the culture's power to distort body image. Even less has been taught to professionals about how to directly encourage kids to be less obsessed about the way they look. Here are several ways that are useful to both professionals and parents:

1. Compliment kids on their unique style. Every time a child goes against the crowd, she needs to be recognized for her courage. Over time, kids can be gently pushed to build on their own unique fashion style. Some feel comfortable *not* wearing designer clothes; some prefer their own taste rather than the crowd's; some take joy in surprise, others in subtlety. Whatever their preferences, in these hyperconscious times, the ability to look different often gives children the strength to act differently than the popular, trendsetting group.

For example, 11-year-old Sue, a slightly gawky and big-boned girl, dressed neither preppy nor laid back. As she experimented with unique looks, a tuned-in teacher, Lisa, was sure to comment when she felt Sue had made a successful "fashion statement." Lisa explained to me that she'd learned over the years to give kids a positive nudge in the direction of forging their own styles.

---

*Margo Maine, *Father Hunger* (Gurze Books, 1991).

A guidance counselor working in a suburban school taught me the following helpful series of questions that gets kids to reflect on their looks, rather than blindly follow trends; using questions such as these, this astute counselor was able to help kids put into words vague feelings of self-consciousness:

- What are you trying to say?
- Who are you trying to be like?
- Who will be mean to you if you dress differently?
- Who will accept you anyway?

2. Go with a child's natural look. Over time adults can help children create an image of themselves that's built on who they truly are. A slightly heavyset child is a lot better off wearing clothes that are flattering to a bigger child rather than launching a rigid diet. A child with "big" ears can be encouraged to find the right hair length or hairstyle that doesn't accentuate the size or shape of his ears. Especially thin kids can wear horizontal stripes to appear more substantial. The solution is less important than *trying*. Kids need to know what they can *do* about their looks. Research shows that action positively affects the nagging self-doubt that lurks for many kids just beneath the surface.

Counselors and teachers I've interviewed in different school settings strike the same note—professionals must notice what makes kids look good and feel natural. In many interviews, kids have commented to me how much they care when important adults flatter them on subtle changes in their hairstyle or the clothes they choose. Kids especially remember comments made about "a look" that is pleasing yet requires very little effort. For example, 14-year-old Jimmy, who felt extremely self-conscious about being a bit overweight, paid attention to his teacher's comments on clothes that were subdued and more subtle than his usual wild tee-shirts and neon pants. Over time, Jimmy started to dress in a more casual way that called less attention to his size; he also was more generally comfortable with himself, participating in class and fitting in better with peers.

3. Limit a child's access to the pop culture. I can tell by the level of a child's obsession over appearance just how much TV she watches and pop magazines she reads. Because of this, there is perhaps no other strategy more important to body image and general self-esteem than limiting access to pop culture. The average number of hours a TV set is on in any given household across the United States each day is approximately 7! Kids of all ages watch 3–5 hours a day. More than 50% of children now have TV sets in their own rooms and, worse, given a choice of being with TV and being with their fathers, a majority will choose TV—a figure that is disturbing although not surprising to professionals who work with families (Kaiser Family Foundation Report, *Kids and Media*, 1999; The Center for Media Education, 1999).

Teachers and educators can help parents draw the line by "strongly suggesting" parameters for "how much is too much," and what parents can do to soften TV's negative effects. Helpful suggestions have been made by the American Pediatric Association and also can be found in the Kaiser Family Foundation's report cited above. The following are some of the most important suggestions:

- The American Pediatric Association suggests that children watch no more than 1–2 hours per day of TV.
- Parents should not allow kids to have media access in their own bedrooms. TV and video games "in the room" lead to higher media use.
- Limit the amount of time that the TV set is on in the home *for everyone,* especially if it's just on as background noise.
- Remind parents that kids watch TV programs, not TV. This begins to teach the idea that kids and parents must make choices about which programs to view.
- Strongly encourage parents to sit with their children and watch programs so as to help the whole family make informed choices. This is just as important for video games, music, and Internet chat rooms.
- Establish rituals that provide togetherness, not reliance on pop culture consumption.
- Explain the *business* of celebrity and beauty—bring into schools models and athletes who can tell the real story behind celebrity.

*   *   *

It is fitting to end a chapter on self-esteem in the 21st century with the topic of kids' exposure to the media. There is a widespread feeling among both parents and professionals that our kids' sense of themselves is affected by pop culture forces that adults can't control. Remembering some of the suggestions offered here can, however, help the grown-ups in children's lives keep priorities clear. There are many pathways to low self-esteem in children, but there is a growing body of knowledge about strengthening a child's resilience. By focusing on the points raised in this chapter, professionals working with families can help kids become more interested in mastery than in consumption, put aside more time to play than to watch, learn how to think realistically rather than obsess, and expect praise only for true effort. These changes can go a long way toward building more resilient self-esteem in our kids.

chapter nine

The Power of Two

Helping Parents Create
a United Front

Many times, when mothers and fathers approach us about difficulties with kids, the hidden item on the agenda is conflict between the parents about how to handle child rearing in a united manner. Yet, creating this elusive united front often turns out to be a greater challenge than it first appears. Something always seems to get in the way of parents agreeing. Most of us have been taught that these conflicts are the result of differences in upbringing. Parents grow up in homes with very different belief systems and must learn the elusive art of compromise for the good of creating a unified message.

Unfortunately, these traditional explanations don't seem to work—parents often continue to disagree in the heat of the moment; they can't see eye to eye, and kids end up slipping through the cracks. Over the years, I began to understand that something far more fundamental creates conflict on the parenting team. Through extensive case reviews, I've come to believe that most parenting struggles are about implicit gender arrangements, which are so personal and culturally ingrained that in order to understand this better I had to take an honest look at gender role definitions in my own upbringing.

This chapter reflects work done with families in my role as a counselor, seen through the lens of my own history as well as the clients I've worked with. From both perspectives, we learn how gender definitions around the house—what mothers and fathers are supposed to do—affect this most elusive of goals: the united front. Along with personal and clinical examples, as in every other chapter, I have included concrete strategies that can be used by any professional who must help parents get on the same wavelength—teachers, counselors, clergy, and so on.

*   *   *

It's 1959, and I have just turned 13. Yet, even as adolescence dawns and I begin to engage in timeless male initiation rites, I can still feel my mother's presence everywhere.

My friend Mark and I are going fishing for the first time with "the men." We are to get up at 4:30 A.M., announces my mother, after getting off the phone with Mark's mother. Deep-sea fishing, I marvel, not quite realizing that the huge marlin I picture valiantly hauling in is actually flounder and the deep sea happens to be a couple of miles off Coney Island.

The next morning before dawn, my mother wakes me up, prepares a big breakfast for my dad and me, and waves goodbye as we trudge out, carrying the lunch she made, along with extra socks and sweaters she packed, in case there is rough surf. Twelve hours later, we wolf down the two tiny flounder my mother has scraped, cleaned, and thoroughly disinfected. Unfortunately, by the time Monday rolls around, I'm in bed, nauseated and blistered from the sun. "Oh, well, it was worth it," I think, as my mother places a cold cloth on my head, and a 7-Up, glass of ice cubes, and her work number next to my bed.

Dennis and Sabrina: A Postliberation Family

It's now more than 40 years later, and the world has turned upside down. Everything, especially the gender landscape, has completely changed . . . well, perhaps not as much as we would like to believe. Dennis, a college instructor, and Sabrina, a corporate executive, come to see me about their 5-year-old son, Lee. Both Dennis and Sabrina have been married before, both are well-paid professionals, both doubted they would have any more children. Dennis informs me, with no small amount of pride, that he is "deeply involved" in his son's upbringing and does a host of household and child-rearing tasks. He plays with his son almost every day, takes him to the park and playground at least once each weekend, and willingly "baby-sits" when Sabrina has to stay late at the office. But even with all his efforts, he complains that they are arguing so badly about how to handle their son that they rarely speak to each other except to fight.

When I ask them what the trouble is, Dennis answers immediately that Lee is having almost daily tantrums. "He isn't making friends in school and alienates a lot of the other kids," Dennis continues. Since Dennis has initiated the conversation and seems so articulate about his son's difficulties, I ask him for more specific details. How does Lee react when he has to share one of his toys?

"Well, ah . . . um . . . he doesn't like it," stammers Dennis, "but I'm not exactly sure just what happens." At this point, Sabrina, who has begun tapping her fingers on her chair, breaks in. "I take him for most of his play dates," she says crisply, and then provides a detailed description of Lee's behavior—how he hoards toys and cries uncontrollably when other children reach for them, how he suddenly develops a passion for any toy that another child is playing with, and so on.

I address a second question to Dennis. "What happens when you're fixing dinner and Lee throws a tantrum? How do you control it? Does a snack help?"

"Well, maybe . . . sometimes . . ., " Dennis says, glancing at Sabrina. "Do you always give him a snack?" he asks her, tentatively.

Sabrina sighs. "Dennis teaches three nights a week and has student office hours on another night, so actually I'm home with Lee most evenings and make dinner for him," she says. "Yes, sometimes a snack calms him down, and sometimes I can distract him by letting him help me with some little thing, like carrying cups to the table. But other times, nothing works at all."

I press on, this time addressing the question to both of them. "What does Lee's teacher say about the trouble he has with his classmates?" As if by mutual consent, Sabrina now takes over. "The teacher believes that Lee has a particularly hard time with two of the rougher boys, Ken and Justin. They are a lot bigger than Lee is and are always bugging him."

"Now, are they the boys who . . . ?" Dennis begins to ask in a puzzled tone.

"I've already told you this, Dennis," Sabrina snaps. "They are the same boys who pushed him into a corner and took his lunch last week."

The "Mom's In Charge, Dad Helps Out" Paradigm

Overall, the meeting sounded exactly like a thousand others I've conducted with families in which a father was "very involved" in raising the child, not only in his own view but often according to his wife as well. Certainly, Dennis was doing much more child care and household work than his father had ever dreamed of doing, and he was much more involved than many of his own peers at work. But if I wanted to know specific details about Lee's life—how he spent his day, how he behaved, where, when, and under what circumstances he had his good times and bad, how his peers and teachers interacted with him—I would have to ask his mother, just as the family pediatrician would have had to ask my mother about me 40 years ago.

However involved Dennis thought he was, however much he and his wife believed they embodied a new 1990s consciousness of "shared parenting," it was obviously still mother who was "parenting central." Sabrina not only carried the lion's share of the physical and practical parenting and housekeeping chores but made most of the daily decisions about Lee's life as well. Nor is this presumably enlightened family uncommon. In spite of massive changes in gender relations over the past 30 years, when children are born, most parents revert to a modified style of traditional parenting, which sociologist Arlie Hochschild referred to as the "Mom's responsible, Dad helps out" paradigm in her widely acclaimed book, *The Second Shift: Working Parents and the Revolution at Home* (Viking Penguin, 1989). According to Hochschild's studies, fathers still are defined, and define themselves, primarily as breadwinners and providers, and only secondarily as "helpers" on the home front. And, in spite of the undeniable changes in fatherhood, compared with the standard 1950s and 1960s model that most young parents remember from their own childhoods, Hochschild estimates that the mothers married to these men do far more housework and parenting than the fathers do—the equivalent of a full month of 24-hour days more than their spouses.

Many years after the book's publication, Hochschild's view is harder to accept. After all, the media—movies, TV sitcoms, magazines—have portrayed a slew of New Age dads handling babies, cooking (or ordering take-out) and advising their preteen youngsters on peer relations and dating strategies. According to a 1993 survey of several hundred parents by *Child* magazine, only 1 in 10 dads considers himself (or is considered by his wife) to be a relatively uninvolved "backseat dad." A full 25% of today's fathers, compared to just 2% a generation ago, regularly participate in the hands-on care of their children—bathing, dressing, diapering, putting to bed, and so on. Unfortunately, in the glow of this progress, it is easy to forget that at the other end of that 25% is the 75% of dads who rarely help out at all. In fact, half of the fathers surveyed who defined their participation at home as "well rounded" meant that they helped with child care only "as their schedules permitted."

The unsettling results in *Child* magazine, with its sample of self-selected and relatively upscale families, could easily be dismissed. However, they are supported by other, more widely based studies. In 1993, the Family and Work Institute conducted a national survey of nearly 3,000 randomly selected men and women cutting across economic, regional, racial, and age groups. Their findings: In postmodern, postfeminist United States, women were still 2 times more likely to pay household bills than men, 5 times more likely to cook for the family, 7 times more likely to do the family shopping, and 11 times more likely to do the household cleaning. This is true, the survey concluded, "even in families where women contribute half or more of the family income and where workers are young." More recent studies show only slight improvement over these highly unbalanced arrangements.

Discovering the Endless List

The continued imbalance between surface appearances and the true nature of daily life needs to be recognized in the couples we meet. Discovering what I call "the endless list" opens the way to a more equitable distribution of child care, and begins the work of creating a true united front. Here's how:

Asking Couples to Record Who Does What

Since there is such a discrepancy between the appearance of change and what actually happens behind closed doors and because I believe hidden imbalances in child care contribute enormously to tension between parents, I've begun asking couples to document who does what around the house. For example, at the end of the first meeting, I asked Dennis and Sabrina to write down everything each of them did or thought about in relation to the kids during a weekday evening or morning. At the next session, they brought their lists, covering a Wednesday night from 6 to 11 P.M. As Dennis's record showed, he *was* involved: calling home to see whether he should pick up anything, setting the dinner table, cleaning up around the house, checking on homework, and reading and saying goodnight to the kids. Dennis, indeed, seemed to be a hands-on father until Sabrina produced *her* list.

Whereas Dennis had recorded a dozen tasks on a 3 × 5 index card, she unfurled a 6-foot scroll that covered almost 100 items. Reading them took the entire session. The following are only a sample: respond to kids badgering her about arrangements for the weekend and asking for permission about snacks; pack bags for sleep-overs; pay bills; call other parents to set up play dates; braid her daughter's hair; make about 20 phone calls as class mother; buy Christmas presents for the baby-sitter; do a load of washing; talk to her husband's mother (after he hands the phone to her); check the kids' homework, feed the cat; write thank-you notes for a recent birthday party.

Sabrina's list seemed truly endless. Her words upon finishing were, "Everything in this family gets routed through me. There isn't a single event that I'm not somehow directly or indirectly involved with. No wonder I walk around feeling exhausted and furious." Even Dennis was taken aback by this graphic evidence of just how unbalanced the division of labor really was in his modern, two-career family. Dennis's quite respectable contributions were little more than footnotes to the vast text of his wife's obligations and tasks, the endless list of parenting demands that mothers typically fulfill.

I've repeated this "endless list" exercise with hundreds of couples, with generally the same result. Not only are both spouses surprised at the discrepancy (fathers are usually stunned), but counselors themselves can get a graphic picture of just how durable the "Mom's responsible, Dad helps out" paradigm is.

Specific Questions That Uncover the Endless List

If you are with parents, ask them the following questions as a gauge of who assumes ultimate responsibility for thinking about the tasks that make up the endless list and seeing that they get done. Since this paradigm is so embedded in all of us, ask yourself as well—who in *your* house knows more of the answers?

1. What are the shoe sizes of your children?
2. Who first notices the signs that one of your children is getting sick?
3. Who informs the school when your child won't be coming and calls the parents of your child's playmates to warn them that she has the chicken pox or some other communicable illness?
4. Who bought the last book on any aspect of child rearing?
5. Who usually buys small "thinking of you" presents when your child seems to be blue?
6. Who sets up play dates, makes the arrangements for them, and thinks ahead about how to schedule the weekend?

7. Who researches local pediatricians, baby-sitters, nursery schools, day care centers, camps, and after-school activities?
8. Who plans and organizes birthday parties and other special child-related events, wraps presents, writes cards, and thank-you notes?
9. Whose date book contains the times of the school concert, Little League sign up, school committee meetings, and other child-related events?
10. Who does your child usually open up to when upset, run to when hurt, or scream at when mad?

If your own household arrangements do not significantly differ from those of most American families in just about any configuration, you, too, have implicitly accepted the standard paradigm of "Mom's responsible, Dad helps out." And this still-taken-for-granted division of labor has profound effects on the parents we meet as well as on our personal lives. For however rationalized, it inevitably generates parental disagreements about child rearing, particularly discipline, communication with kids, and life-cycle transitions, the very subjects that often bring families to seek our help.

Discipline and the Endless List

When it came to "the rules," my mother and I engaged in daily guerrilla warfare. It was amazing how many brush fires could begin and then abruptly die out in that half-hour before my father arrived. There seemed to be no end to the chores I was supposed to do, all of which I wheedled, debated, and tried to cajole my way out of—until the inevitable "Wait until your father gets home!" If things hadn't gone well for him at work and the squabbling at home continued, he'd erupt in a rage. And yet, while his volcanic anger was frightening, it seemed curiously disconnected from my daily life, a distant thunderclap as my mother and I trudged through the swamp of family routine.

Why Dads Often Seem "Tougher"

However placid a family appears, however well behaved the children, chances are that beneath the surface there are numerous arguments between the parents about discipline. "He's too rough—he won't give the kid a chance to explain before lighting into him like a tough cop," complains Mom. "She's such a marshmallow—she just lets the kids walk all over her," Dad rejoins. Traditionally, men have been regarded as "tough-minded" and "dispassionate," while women are considered more "empathic" and "sensitive," viewing their children through a rosy lens of "mother love" and therefore seen as less effective disciplinarians. In the classical era of family therapy, clinicians implicitly reinforced this notion with interventions designed to create "more appropriate" hierarchies within families. We encouraged mothers to move offstage, while we brought in fathers' more "realistic" ways of parenting.

I now believe that women's responsibility for fulfilling the demand of the endless list turns this stereotype upside down. Men, insulated from the chaos of daily life with children, protected from the constant pressure to plan and carry through the details of child rearing, can afford the luxury of disciplinary idealism, whereas women quickly learn the necessity of hard-nosed pragmatism—if they want to survive emotionally and see their children grow up. As keepers of tradition, men can create disciplinary scenarios of perfect fairness and justice. Women, on the other hand, struggle day to day in the trenches. They must learn to accept little defeats to avoid bigger ones, settle for imperfect victories, and learn the fine art of creative haggling.

The "Mom's responsible, Dad helps out" paradigm showed up during a heated exchange between Michelle and Howard, the parents of 4-year-old Lydia, while they were attending one of my parenting workshops. The couple had taken Lydia to a concert, a 2-hour affair that had clearly outstripped the child's capacity for decorum, patience, and music appreciation. Between periods of relative quiet, her squirming and whining aggravated Howard so much that even the memory of it caused him to yell at his wife in front of 200 other workshop attendees: "She disturbed everybody within earshot! She was awful! And you just let it go on! If we don't make her behave now, how will she ever learn to sit still and be quiet?"

Michelle, no more intimidated by 200 other parents than by Howard, yelled back, "What the hell do you want from a 4-year-old? She hadn't had a nap, she had practically no lunch, and she's a very little girl. At least we got through the entire concert, and she only really started having trouble at the end." What fueled Michelle's argument was, first, her practical knowledge, borne of experience, that Lydia had not been so bad (all things considered, it was unlikely, short of using terrorist tactics, that they could transform their active 4-year-old into an ideal concertgoer); and, second, the realistic belief that if Lydia created a scene in front of a crowd, she, as the mother, would be held responsible by everybody there.

Helping the "Pragmatist" and the "Idealist" Agree

Ironically, when it comes to discipline, the pragmatist versus the idealist split often occurs in the other direction as well, with the mother becoming the family authoritarian, while the father assumes the role of humanitarian and all-around nice guy. "I feel like a drill sergeant," I've heard thousands of mothers say, "but if I don't keep pushing, pushing, pushing, the kids won't get to school on time, homework and chores won't get done, dinner will never be on the table, nobody will ever get to bed." And in the face of what these mothers feel is an uphill battle to keep the household from falling into total chaos, fathers often get in the way: "He never sets any limits. He goes behind my back and lets them do things I've told them they can't do—the way he turns me into the heavy makes me sick." To which Dad typically retorts, "She's much too rigid; she makes a federal case out of every little thing they do. I don't see why she's so controlling—they're really pretty good kids."

Is this still Mom as pragmatist and Dad as idealist? Absolutely. She feels she is barely treading water, overwhelmed by demands and duties, required to come down hard on the kids (and Dad) in order to keep a thin veneer of control over the potential chaos that

American family life often resembles. "Mr. Nice Guy," on the other hand, can maintain his good nature precisely because he is spared just enough of the struggle and organizational responsibility to keep his cool. How do you help parents get past these profoundly ingrained beliefs so they can be a more united team? The indirect route of addressing the endless list is the way to proceed. Follow these steps:

1. **Ask about the endless list.** Jim, an even-tempered father, for example, complained about the screaming around the house every morning: "I can't stand the struggles between Sally and the children—she's on their case from the minute they get up. I can't believe this is the way the day has to start. Why burden them with so many rules and 'shoulds'?" "He's right," his wife, Sally said, near tears, "I'm impossible. I can't stand myself either."

When I asked how the morning worked and who did what with the kids, the reasons for Sally's "impossibility" became more clear. She began to describe the morning chaos: brushing teeth, getting washed, finding the right clothes, fixing lunch, dealing with unexpected tantrums, and so on. Many of these tasks were evenly divided—except for one small detail: somehow, Jim was allowed 30 extra minutes in the bathroom to prepare for the workday. During those precious 30 minutes, it was up to Sally to get the kids finished dressing, make sure they had their homework, referee last-minute quarrels, and get herself ready for work as well. This uneven distribution of a vital commodity—time—was taken for granted by both spouses. Jim might have been Mr. Nice Guy and Sally too driven, but behind her tension was a hard-boiled pragmatist trying to make a dent in the endless list. "Things have to get done by a certain time. Otherwise, the school bus will leave without Becky or the lunches won't be packed, or . . . or . . . " Somebody had to think about these things, but it wasn't going to be Jim, at least not during his half-hour meditation in the bathroom.

2. **Get Mom and Dad to briefly change roles.** I asked Sally and Jim to change roles for just one or two mornings, allowing her an extra 30 minutes alone while he launched the kids on their

morning routine. At first, Sally refused. Like many mothers, she felt uneasy about relinquishing control and was afraid Jim wouldn't get it right: "I know what to do—I can handle it. Besides, the kids will want me anyway. Let's just leave things the way they are." I encouraged her to let Jim deal with the kids when they started screaming "I want Mommy." Finally, she agreed she would try to ignore their pleas and ride her exercise bike for 30 minutes while he took on this added section of the endless list. For both Jim and Sally, the experience was a revelation. "I was awful," he admitted, now sounding as self-critical as his wife. "They drove me crazy. I got furious. I yelled, I screamed, I threatened. I did anything I could to get them going and out of the house on time. And I ended up being late to work anyway."

3. Encourage Dad to talk to kids directly before decisions are made. The idealist father and the pragmatist mother are often needlessly pitted against each other if only Mom has the details regarding specific upcoming events. If you encourage Dad to speak directly to a child on a kind of fact-finding mission, more often than not his approach upon hearing the details immediately becomes more pragmatic. For example, in one family I met, there was a great deal of arguing between Peter and Louise about their two young adolescent daughters. Almost always, Peter was on the side of being tougher and more restrictive toward the kids. Mom would be caught in the middle, usually having spoken to the children and also to other parents. This particular fight was around an upcoming party that one of the girls, Dana, wanted to attend. Peter took his usual stricter stance, while Mom was more at ease. So I asked Peter to speak directly to Dana instead of armchair quarterbacking with Mom. As Peter and Dana discussed the details of supervision of the party—who was going to be there, when and how Dana would get home—Peter gradually eased up on his theoretical position. Just this one conversation illustrated to both parents how important it was to maintaining a united front that Peter speak more often to his daughters. The number of disagreements between Louise and Peter sharply diminished after Peter got more involved.

Balanced participation is the great equalizer. As long as mothers are still implicitly in charge of the endless list, their disciplinary approach is often based on the pragmatic belief that "I just want to get through the day. If it works, I'll use it." From this perspective, it matters little whether a father is strict but continues to emphasize character-building discipline or whether he is lenient and stresses the necessity of teaching independent thought; he might as well be talking a foreign language to the overloaded pragmatist he lives with. He is ultimately dismissed by both mother and child. This is less because of any chronic pathological dynamics within the house, as classic family therapy tradition might have diagnosed it, than because he has not put in enough time on the endless list to give him the legitimacy to claim true authority.

Communication and the Endless List

I was 16 and sitting in the living room, crushed that my girlfriend was breaking up with me. I hardly noticed my mother somewhere nearby, on her weekly search-and-destroy mission against lint, dust, grease, and grime—all of which she could (with some justification) trace back to me. Without looking over her shoulder, she said, "Ronnie, is something wrong?" Tears formed tiny rivulets down my cheeks. I mumbled, without looking up, "Laura is breaking . . . " She stopped for a moment, put her hand on my shoulder, and said, softly, "Well, there'll be others. You'll see."

Although not exactly high-tech parenting, something about this tender cliche made me feel just a little bit better. By the time my father came home 20 minutes later, I was still feeling bad but certainly would never mention it again. In our family, this kind of deep, interpersonal exchange was a rare event—and you just had to be there at the right time.

Why Kids Talk More to Mothers

A tragic imbalance in family life is that children usually open up more to mothers than to fathers. Longitudinal research on normal families has long demonstrated this, as does my own clinical experience with dysfunctional families. But 15-year-old Bobby put it best: "My dad and I have a real strong father–son thing, but I save the important, emotional stuff for my mom."

Kids Talk while Engaged in Ordinary Tasks

Again, one can lean on stereotypes for explanations. After all, women are socialized to be good listeners, to be empathic, sensitive, etc., and so it makes sense for children to seek them out. However, in daily life there is a more ordinary reason why kids don't communicate as readily with fathers. As I've described in Chapter 10, no child of any age opens up according to a predictable schedule; kids talk when and where they feel like it, usually while carrying out parallel, mindless activities with a parent. Consequently, the parent who engages in more drudgery with children, who sets a dinner table with them, puts them to bed, gives them a bath, goes to the doctor, wraps presents, or drives them to their activities is *the one who learns the facts of their lives*. Obviously, when the endless list is imbalanced, communication is out of kilter as well, because one parent (usually the mother) gets more of the exposure. The stage is set for Mom to become the child expert and for Dad to slip away from the family's emotional center and eventually find himself at the periphery of its daily life.

The interactive fluidity that develops between mothers and children is secretly envied by many fathers even when they criticize their partners. Laird, for example, complained about his wife Harriet's short temper. Still, he also envied the way she and their two grade-school children interacted so effortlessly. Laird described the following scene:

MOM: Hurry up and get dressed. You're going to miss the bus.

BOBBY: My toast is burned. I don't want to eat it.

AMY: Mom, Bobby took my hairbrush again!

MOM (*more loudly*): Will you both stop dawdling and get moving!

BOBBY: I was only going to use it for 5 minutes.

MOM: Amy, did you wash your face?

AMY: (*Doesn't answer, stares at the TV.*)

MOM (*yelling*): Amy, I said did you wash up? Bobby, I don't see you putting your socks on!

AMY: Mom, stop screaming. I'm tired. I don't want to put my clothes on yet.

MOM (*screaming*): I've had it with you two! Get downstairs right this very minute or . . . !

Yet, five minutes after this series of miniexplosions, Bobby is contentedly sitting next to Mom munching cereal and Amy is on Mom's lap getting her hair brushed as if nothing had happened. Laird may be right to worry about these scenes; Harriet and the kids are probably embroiled in too many power struggles. At the same time, he feels like a spectator watching another species in their natural habitat, and there is something pained in his voice as he describes these strange beings who inhabit his house. They are the family, he almost feels, while he is not quite part of it.

When Dads Don't do the Drudge Work, Kids Don't Talk

If drudgery is the glue of everyday life, then details are its active ingredients. When a father doesn't know the names of the children in his daughter's class, or exactly which kids compose the "in" group and which compose the "out" group; when he isn't in direct communication with the teacher about absences or schoolwork, vague questions like "How was school today?" end up being met with maddeningly opaque answers. The stonewalling that kids do (to both parents) can especially hurt fathers who already feel peripheral to the life of the family.

Speaking for many, Perry, a dad in a parenting workshop, asked his 9-year-old son, John, "Why don't you give me a straight answer when I ask you about school? I'm tired of hearing everything from your mother. It really bothers me."

"But you don't ask specific questions," John articulately replied. "When you say, 'How was school today?' I don't know what you mean. If you were more specific, I'd remember better. It makes me think you're not really interested."

John's words plunged 100 parents and children into total silence. You could feel sadness spreading across the room. This classic misunderstanding between a father and child is incredibly familiar. Perry does care—it was impossible to miss the hurt look on his face. But his inability to ask precise, detailed questions caused John to doubt his sincerity, his authentic desire to know. Like too many fathers, Perry ends up feeling rejected. He subtly withdraws, then must rely even more on his wife for information, while increasingly resenting her position as family switchboard. In the meantime, she feels indispensable but increasingly overwhelmed.

Challenging Fathers to Take on More of the Endless List—Ordinary, Child-Maintenance Tasks

Besides mothers feeling overwhelmed and resentful, the single biggest source of disconnection in family life is fathers feeling hurt and left out. A lot of abusive or harsh fathers do so because that's their way of barging in. An example was a couple I know in which Sid, the father, would scream at the kids. Regarding a specific incident, I asked Sid, "Why did you yell at your 4-year-old and then rip him out of the car seat?" Sid replied, "Because the entire car ride, my kid kept talking to my wife, even though I was doing all the driving after a week of hard work. I felt like I just didn't exist."

Men's solution to this peripherality is to engage in "Mr. Excitement" activities. Unfortunately, as a way to connect, these events usually don't work. Children do not bond during a ride on a roller coaster, or when "the wave" goes through a ballpark. Kids often don't even remember who took them to such megacharged events. Instead, kids connect during the times that are ordinary and comforting—the in-between moments: homework, getting through the evening grind, hanging out watching TV. The kids I've interviewed repeatedly say these are the times that matter. The more you can encourage fathers to take on those comforting low-key responsibilities, the more they will feel bonded to their children.

Think small. For example, a couple, Alice and Tom, who came to me had not had sex for 2 years. Gabby, their child, was 4½ years old. Alice and Tom were obviously becoming more disconnected from each other and frequently fighting. I asked them to do the "endless list" exercise, which uncovered an interesting detail: every morning their Gabby went over to Alice's side of the bed and said, "Mommy, fix me some Lucky Charms." Alice, thinking only *she* could do it, would always get up and fix those Lucky Charms. "Why," I asked, "do you have to do it?" And Alice said, "Well, if Tom tries, it won't get done right." I said, "We're talking about Lucky Charms, not open heart surgery!" Of course, as any parent knows, there *are* a million ways to screw up Lucky Charms: too much milk, too little milk, too many charms, the wrong bowl, the wrong spoon. And, predicting difficulty, as we should with all parents—it's not like Gabby will love this change and say, "Oh great, Dad's going to do it!" Mom accurately warned, "I'll say no, but Gabby will refuse and insist, 'No, I want *you* to do it, Mommy!' "— I, as always, searched for the point of just-tolerable change: "Alright, then don't do it often. Let's agree that you'll try it once during the next couple of weeks." We finally agreed to "once this month."

So they came back later that month, and Gabby had indeed resisted: "No, not Daddy, I want Mommy to do it!" But Alice said something that was, for her family, very revolutionary: "No, *I* want to sleep longer. *I'm* tired. *I* need some rest, Sweetie. Wake Daddy up!" Gabby *did* wake Tom up; he stumbled out and fixed the Lucky Charms. Of course, Daddy "got it all wrong." But it was just good enough. Most important, Alice didn't say anything—she made no "supervisory" comments whatsoever. A week later, Dad took care of the Lucky Charms again. The next week, something truly unexpected happened: at 2:45 in the morning, Gabby woke up sick. All of a sudden she screamed out, "*Daddy*, come here and help me!" Tom went to her, and the next time we met he laughingly said, "I hate you and I love you. I'm not going to pretend I'm thrilled that I had to get up in the middle of the night but" (and here's the key phrase) "it was the first time I ever felt that Gabby needed me as much as she needed her mom. It gave me something back; and I wanted to do more." As happens so often, false-self change leads to positive reinforcement and then genuine motivation. This sequence of events was the beginning of greater connection in this couple.

Simple changes can sometimes make enormous differences. For example, Bert knew that his 8-year-old stepson, Charlie, was having trouble at school, but all his information had come second-hand, from his wife, Yvonne. Trying to forge some connection of his own with Charlie, he tried talking to him about school, but to every question all he got were monosyllables. Feeling more than a little rejected, he tried to push his way into the family configuration by second-guessing and criticizing Yvonne, telling her how to discipline Charlie and accusing her of not being "tough enough." Yvonne was furious and counterattacked by calling him a "backseat driver" and told him he had some nerve to lecture her when he didn't have a clue about what was going on. Their fights about child rearing had led them to consider divorce.

I suggested one small change: that Bert take Charlie with him every Saturday and Sunday to get the newspapers—a leisurely 15-minute stroll into town. Both Yvonne and Bert looked as if I were obviously too simple minded to be engaged with the complex job of helping a stepfamily. "Give me a break!" said Yvonne. "You don't seriously believe that will make a difference?" Bert asked in disbelief. But they tried it, and 2 weeks later, on one of their newspaper strolls, Charlie started telling Bert that he had become the class scapegoat. He finished his fairly long recitation by asking, a little timidly, whether Bert might have some advice for him on how to handle the situation. This was the first satisfying conversation Bert had had with his stepson since the two met.

Mothers Need to Stop Monitoring

What I hear from men all over the country is strikingly consistent: "She wants me to do half the work; but she has to stop supervising and criticizing how I handle things." When mothers are really honest, many admit to this, offering the plea of "guilty with an explanation": "If I don't do the job, it won't get done right," or, "If I don't take charge, it's simply not going to get done." Whenever you hear such descriptions, the "Mom's in charge, Dad helps out" paradigm is at work and you need to challenge these beliefs.

Push mothers to face their anxiety about letting go. Say, "You need to try once a week not to criticize or supervise something he does." Then search for the just-tolerable level of anxiety: "You can't do it once a week? Try once very other week . . . " After a goal has been reached, the following phrase provides motivation to help anxious mothers let go: "Ask yourself, Mom, what's more important—that it's done 'right' or that he develops a stronger connection with the kids?" In most situations (excluding, of course, any that may result in physical danger), overwhelmed mothers opt for a "stronger connection" between father and their children. The choice between perfectly coifed kids in the morning pales by comparison to a more involved partner.

Bert and Charlie's 15-minute walk addressed three complex problem areas: first, it allowed them to connect without Yvonne as the intermediary; second, Yvonne and Bert fought less about who was the real child-rearing "expert"; third, the new connection with Charlie felt so good to Bert that he figured out other ways to spend ordinary time with him. Within four sessions, the fighting between Yvonne and Bert significantly lessened and all three were beginning to feel like a real family.

Getting Moms to *Not* Thank Dads for What They Do

Many women in interviews are quite blunt: "Let's face it, most men need appreciation; men have to be acknowledged—they're such babies." Fathers believe that they should be thanked for contributions. While we've found appreciation to be essential, we've also found is that it should be for the right reason. "Thanks, Dad, for helping me out," keeps the "Mom's in charge" paradigm intact. Every time Mom says that, Dad feels thanked but viewed as an assistant to the real boss—Mom.

The more we challenge this supervisor–apprentice model, the

greater the chance of creating a mutually respectful friendship between parents. And, in fact, every couple interviewed in our study told us that mutual respect was essential to a better relationship and the mood of the household.

*   *   *

When I was 17, the law, in its infinite wisdom, permitted me, as a high-school senior, to drive a two-ton Chevrolet around town. This transition did not bode well for peace in the Taffel household. In my parents' vivid but not unrealistic mutual imaginings, there was no end to the trouble that could happen in the immediate vicinity of the car, not to mention the mischief that might occur inside it. So, returning late at night, I inevitably found my mother hanging out the window, poised to dial the police emergency number. Unaware that she was fronting for the real worrier, my father, sparks flew between us because of this humiliating display of overprotectiveness.

One particular night after I drove off, it started snowing. Not surprisingly, when I returned home, there she was at the window. I went to their bedroom to engage in the old-fashioned custom of kissing my parents goodnight and found her in bed, pretending to be asleep. "Oh," she said, in a feigned, dreamy voice. "Did you just get home?" She did this so convincingly that I began to think I had imagined seeing her at the window—except that her hair was wet and sprinkled with unmelted snow.

Family Transitions and the Endless List

Discipline and communication are not the only issues affected by the "Mom's responsible, Dad helps out" paradigm. Imbalances in the endless list also sow seeds for explosive differences during important developmental transitions, which are the times when professionals most often meet families. Once again, the "Mom's responsible, Dad helps out" paradigm is usually ignored by us. But the imbalance in child-rearing expectations practically guarantees that women and men enter these impending transitions at very different points in time—Mom several months to years earlier than Dad. There are several reasons why:

1. Mothers are usually responsible for transitions. If mothers are in charge of the family's everyday emotional life, they are held particularly responsible for managing family change and child development. By the time Dad realizes that Jimmy is crawling and follows him around with a camera to catch every precious moment, Mom has long since begun thinking about how to baby-proof the house. Indeed, she has probably spoken to her own mother or sister, consulted other mothers, or read magazines on the subject and made plans for the contents of all lower-level cupboards and drawers.

In one family, Marlon, the father, demanded of his wife, Rhona, "Why can't you just say goodnight and leave?" Their younger son, Alex, is 6 months old, and they came to see me because the intimacy in their relationship (a second marriage for both) had dipped to what they consider to be a dangerously low level. Marlon goes on, "It takes you an hour to get ready to leave the house—and we'll only be gone for a couple of hours anyway. You just can't let go. You're more interested in Alex than me!"

Marlon lays the problem directly at Rhona's feet; he thinks she wants nothing to do with him, and he's begun to slip defensively toward the periphery, working extra hours, coming home later, and participating less at home. But, if we look at Rhona's behavior from the "endless list" perspective, maybe she isn't just another overinvolved mother who is ignoring her mate. Perhaps she is checking to make sure there are enough diapers and bottles for the baby, showing the baby-sitter where cookies and chips are stored in case she gets hungry, writing down emergency numbers, instructing the baby-sitter about what to do if Alex has trouble getting to sleep, and taking a little extra time to make sure she and her child feel comfortable with this relative stranger. Meanwhile, Marlon sits out in the car, fuming. But, as loving and committed a father as he is, he doesn't feel responsible for the transition. Therefore, he doesn't experience direct involvement with the details. Instead, he feels hurt and aggravated because Rhona is ignoring him.

2. Mothers have inside information about transitions. Another reason women and men are out of synch during transitions is because mothers have more inside information about what's really going on—and with kids today there's plenty to worry about. Cliff and Beatrice, parents of 14-year-old Marie, came to see me because of their escalating fights over dealing with Marie's push toward independence. This particular argument was about a Friday night party:

> *"Everybody will be there," Marie screamed at her mother. "I'll die if I'm the only one who can't go. Dad said I could go if you say it's OK," she challenged.*
>
> *"Well, it's not OK," Beatrice insisted.*
>
> *"You never want me to have any fun!" Marie accused.*
>
> *Cliff sided with his daughter. "It's just a simple party. You've got to let her grow up," he shouted at his wife.*
>
> *"Maybe I do have a problem letting go," Beatrice said. "But do you know who will be at this party? Did you speak with any of the other parents to find out what's happening?"*

Of course, Cliff hadn't. As it almost always is, the telephone network had been "manned" by women. Having spoken with the other mothers involved, Beatrice knew a few details that Cliff didn't. Indeed, the host parents would not be home; elderly grandparents would be in charge. She also heard talk that some neighborhood kids were going to crash the party with LSD, marijuana, and beer. Cliff cared just as much as Beatrice about his daughter's welfare, and as soon as he learned these details and questioned Marie himself, he changed his position immediately. "Forget it," he said to his daughter, "your mother is right. There isn't enough supervision for my taste either."

3. Mothers are often affected more by family transitions. Mothers and fathers are on separate wavelengths during transitions because their lives are affected in vastly different ways. Each change in a child's routine precipitates losses and beginnings that significantly alter the way mothers concretely live their lives. For example, Joyce, a mother I met at a parenting workshop, described how she felt the year her daughter began kindergarten: "Jenny had gone to the same preschool for 3 years. I knew all the teachers and many of the other parents. We had a certain routine; I knew which mothers I could depend on. Now, there are all new faces when I drop her off on my way to work. I know it will pass, but right now I feel lost."

Clearly, Joyce was not only letting Jenny go but losing an important support group as well. Her husband, Les, was elated by his daughter's transition to real school and couldn't understand why Joyce was so upset. He suspected that she "just wanted to keep Jenny a baby" and didn't realize that his wife was saying good-bye to a vital network that had been very important to her.

Getting Parents in Synch during Transitions

The subtle threads of professional advice to parents are actually sophisticated ways of helping parents "get into synch" so they can start doing the job together with the same information and in the same time frame. This is easier said than done; there are several key factors that help foster this change:

1. **Getting parents on the same page.** During transitions there are some extremely concrete jobs to be done. Many are so obvious we overlook how critical it is for mothers *not* to be entirely responsible (see the accompanying box).

2. **Stop protecting men.** Women and men both protect men, who often say, "I can't do this because I have to work; my work is my identity. My job is to provide. And I can't be disturbed during work with the details of these changes." I used to buy it. I don't buy it any more (see the accompanying box). Somewhere along the line, I decided in my own life, after working with so many different families, that it was important to tell the new school, for example, "The next time our daughter is homesick, *call me*." Say to men, "Unless you're in the middle of doing brain surgery, you need to do this once, just once, to see what it feels like." Once *is* enough. Kids are so stunned, their gratitude breaks through to Dad—false-self change then becomes real. The first time Albert did this with his daughter, Jamie, she was so stunned, she said, "*You* came? *You* came

Ways Partners Can Stay
Connected during Transitions

Here are a half dozen of the most important areas that ought to be addressed by parents *together*:

1. Partners should read written information about upcoming transitions.
2. Fathers ought to make some of the logistical calls to arrange transitions.
3. Mothers need to instruct schools, camps, and social services to also contact fathers about upcoming changes.
4. Fathers need to be included on search interviews—for, say, pediatricians or baby-sitters.
5. Both parents must visit potential new schools, churches, or community organizations before decisions are made.
6. Both mothers and fathers should check out support networks available in the area.

to school?" And for Albert, that moment was the beginning of change, and a transition in which both partners contributed.

3. Help dads remember good role models. When you challenge dads to become more involved in family transitions, many will say, "I had no role model. I didn't have a father who ever did this stuff." Which is true in a lot of cases. When this happens, say, "I want you to think about one time in your life, just one, when either your father, an uncle, a teacher, a coach—any male figure—was good to you, was kind to you, was comforting to you. I want you to close your eyes and think about what they actually did—helped you out, made a call, talked to a teacher, etc." Almost every time a man is asked to think about that, he starts to cry. After such memories have been triggered, add, "The way you felt then, that's the way your child is going to feel toward you for getting more involved. And this is what you want, isn't it?"

How Child Professionals Can Weaken the United Front

Inadvertently we create divisions between parents when we—

- Send written materials (school reports, meeting dates, etc.) to one house in a divorced family rather than both
- Expect that only Mom will attend to details of meeting time
- Don't take an extra step (phone, e-mail) to make sure fathers are included
- Automatically divide tasks according to stereotypical gender roles—discipline to fathers; comforting and arranging to mothers
- Call only mothers when children become sick in school
- Assume that meetings must be built around father's nonnegotiable business schedules

---

For example, Nicholas was acting up a lot in school. His dad, Robert, came to see me because he was upset about Nicholas's downward spiral in his studies. Though he was worried, Robert had never talked with Nicholas's teacher personally, visited the school, nor attended parent–teacher conferences. Because of this, his effort to help Nicholas was seen by the boy as, at best, peripheral and, at worst, comments by someone who didn't know much about what was really going on. When I suggested to Robert that he call the teacher or visit the school counselor himself, he balked, saying, "Fathers don't do that. Mine never did." At which point I responded, "Someone, whether it was your father or another relative, or a friend—some man in your past must have done something helpful to you. See if you can remember." Robert closed his eyes and within a few seconds vividly recalled how his uncle had once stepped in and protected him from an abusive Little League coach. With tears in his eyes, Robert immediately understood how much it had meant to him and how important it was that he take a more active role with Nicholas.

*   *   *

Therapeutic tasks and interventions that move parents into some kind of healthy synchronicity are all to the good. But no technique, no course on parenting skills, and no authoritative pronouncement of the latest fashionable child-rearing theory can work in the long run if they are not grounded in the fundamental assumption that both parents are ultimately responsible for the endless list of child rearing And this responsibility is expressed in the thousands of mundane, gritty and often boring tasks that constitute the daily grind of good-enough parenting. Paradoxically, recognizing its taken-for-granted ordinariness can set off all kinds of fireworks. So go slowly—you are challenging age-old beliefs, the very fabric of many families' lives, and what many mothers and fathers expect from each other.

*   *   *

Five A.M. on September 10, 1985, I awoke from a dream in which my mother's hand was withering away and she was going to join my father, who had died when I was 22, in another land. "It's just a dream," I thought to myself. I'd spoken to her the day before, and she sounded fine. A bit worried, though, I tried to call her before my first patient. Unfortunately, I got a busy signal.

By 2:30, when I arrived at the hospital, she was dying from a virulent infection of the bloodstream, one organ system shutting down after the other. Three hours later, my mother was dead. I soon learned that her symptoms had started at 5:00 A.M., exactly when I was having that dream.

To explain this extraordinary coincidence, one could hypothesize about our continued unconscious merger, lack of differentiation, or even telepathic communication. Perhaps there's some truth to all of this. But, over the years, I've found another, simpler explanation. It was those hours of ordinary time, her endless list, that got under my skin and into my soul. Even as I looked with horror and disbelief at her lifeless body, I suddenly realized that this was the first time I had ever seen my mother still.

chapter ten

Families Under Siege

Helping Parents
and Children Connect

That modern families are under siege is far from
an overstatement. Between continuing high
rates of divorce, job redefinition and relocation, urban and suburban sprawl, and increased work hours and time spent commuting,
there is much evidence that daily family life is at best frazzled and at
worst fragmented. Economic strain adds to family separateness:
mothers return to the work force earlier and in record numbers;
children begin day care at earlier ages; families usually need two in-
comes just to get by.

In response to family fragmentation, there is growing pressure
from some groups to reassert the traditional roles of women as
nurturers and fathers as breadwinners. This theoretical and politi-
cally based solution to fragmented family living is not always helpful to professionals who deal every day with stark reality pressures
on family life. Yet, the question of how families can become more
connected is an *urgent one*. And, since this guide offers concrete solutions rather than theoretical ones, I will provide answers taken
from clinical sources as well as interviews with "well-functioning"
couples: heterosexual, gay and lesbian, multicultural, etc.

The results from these varied sources were remarkably consistent. Over time I've discovered that the groups, diverse as they may
be, engaged in similar practices to maintain satisfactory levels of connection between family members. Each had independently discov-

ered what was needed to feel less daily pressure and disconnection. From these sources, I have identified the following practices that families need to consider in order to stay connected. All professionals who work with parents and kids should know what they are.

Challenging the "Mom's In Charge, Dad Helps Out" Paradigm

As I discussed in the previous chapter, helping parents become aware of the "Mom's helps out" paradigm is the first and most powerful way professionals can ensure greater family connection. Just think about your own life or the families you work with. When two adults exist hierarchically regarding their children and the household, we have found resentment, less sexual desire, parallel living, or adversarial relationships. Only when we begin to challenge the "Mom's responsible; Dad helps out" paradigm do we begin to realize how deeply ingrained the myth is. The most powerful way to change this invisible belief system is to uncover the "endless list," as we explored in Chapter 9.

One family came to me with very serious problems: the three kids were trashing the house and verbally abusing the parents; both teenage boys were in trouble in school. Isolated from extended family and neighborhood supports, this truly was a family under siege!

After the "endless list" exercise, a basic source of tension was unearthed. Elaine, the mother, was chronically resentful about all she was doing, while Bob, the father, felt minimized regarding his very real contributions. Resentment had taken its toll—the two couldn't even be friends, let alone get on the same wavelength regarding the kids. When Elaine saw all her responsibilities in black and white, she said, "I never realized that every single thing in this house goes through me." And Bob said, "Before this, I never 'got' exactly what it was she was always complaining about."

It's not just mothers who are overwhelmed by rigid role definitions and the endless list. Part of the value of the exercise is concretizing the hidden chores fathers do that kids and mothers often take for granted. For example, Bob's main contributions were the peripheral support activities that aren't often recognized—caring for the car, yard work, and heavy-duty carpentry and repairs around the house. This endless list exercise began a process of renegotiating and eventual healing between Bob and Elaine. Appreciating each other's contribution opened the lines of communication just enough so that they could begin creating a more united front for their troubled children.

Unfortunately, Elaine and Bob had to learn the hard way. Role sharing and appreciation of each other's efforts *is precisely what every one of our well-functioning couples reported in interviews.* Many household tasks were shared, even though they might traditionally have been labeled "male" or "female"; almost all of the men regularly cooked, went shopping, put the kids to bed, gave baths, and so on; most of the women did finances and paid bills, took some responsibility for car maintenance, and certainly disciplined the kids. It is not surprising, therefore, that when Bob and Elaine began reassigning some of the tasks around the house—who put the kids to bed every night, for example—it helped them more feel more like two adults participating on an effective team.

Overscheduling and Family Fatigue Syndrome

One of the areas we take for granted is just how overscheduled and ragged family living is. Of course, if we look at our own lives—rushing to and from work, volunteer committee meetings, taking care of household errands, and so on—it is immediately apparent just how frayed we can become. Since most people we meet do not approach us because of complaints about their busy lives, too often we don't address the pace of living when, in fact, it can be a major contributor to children's problems. Kids, on the other hand, often complain in the workshops I run and the interviews I've done with them that life is simply "too much." The kids are right on target. Disconnection in everyday relationships is a natural result of schedules that sprawl uncontrolled into every corner of family life. That is why it is essential not to ignore the everyday logistics and scheduling that can twist family relationships inside out.

Practically every parent I know complains about being exhausted. Although longer work hours and complicated scheduling grab the headlines, a more subtle factor is how late many of our kids get to bed. Maya, a client of mine and the mother of children ages 4 and 6, summed it up: "Between my own guilt about working and my kids' endless negotiating to stay up later, I end up caving in and let them stay up way too late." When kids can define their own bedtime it often leads to a stressed-out, exhausted family the next day. It's a domino effect: the parents' to-do list gets longer, and they have no time for their partners or themselves.

1. Help parents not let guilt be their guide. Maya needed to understand that working during the day didn't mean she had to grant her children's every request at night. But when she began sounding authoritative and enforcing bedtime, her kids were furious with Mom's new priority. To keep herself from buckling under, she repeated this mantra to herself: "When we're all exhausted, nobody wins."

Maya's determination helped her get better organized. Instead of letting routines pile up, she started the bedtime process earlier and divided it into smaller, supervisable chunks: pajamas right after dinner, washing up an hour later, and reading in bed a half hour after that.

Realizing how much better she and the children felt when they were well rested gave Maya the confidence (back to the endless list) to ask her husband Marty to change his evening patterns too: "I know you want to play with the kids when you come home, but arriving so close to their bedtime gets them too excited to go to sleep." Marty agreed, and within a few days he got permission to leave work 45 minutes earlier twice a week in exchange for working through lunch. "That may not seem like much," Maya said to me, "but for us it was a personal revolution." How do Maya and Marty use their new-found time? They've discovered that even 15 minutes dedicated to themselves—for example, to reading or exercising—goes a long way toward relieving stress and increasing connection.

2. Establish boundaries around the permeable family. Today's family has lost it's distinct boundaries and, along with them,
the ability to relax and often relate. High-tech communication in
the form of cellular phones, e-mail, beepers, and faxes invades the
sanctity—and sanity—of home life, creating households as chaotic
and stressful as a 24-hour shopping mall.

Parents must decide whom they'll accept communication from
and who will need to wait. Of course, whenever you help to set priorities that leave people out, feathers will be initially ruffled. For example, Lisa's mother-in-law, Nadine, always seemed to call at an in-
convenient time, before meals or just when Lisa was finally sitting
down to relax. With my encouragement, Lisa took charge. She explained what the problem was and asked her mother-in-law to
phone around 10 at night. "Nadine was annoyed at first," says Lisa,
"but gradually she got used to the new schedule."

Because Lisa could better focus without interruptions, she got
dragged into few witching-hour and bedtime fights with the kids—
an improvement that significantly lowered everyday friction.

It may also be necessary to literally turn off computers, beepers, and fax lines at night. For example, initially, Tom felt uneasy
telling his colleagues and people he volunteered with that at certain
times he would be unavailable. "But now it's been better around
the house," Tom notes. "Dinnertime is calmer, and I even have
time to read to the kids."

3. Fight perfectionism. If parents are still trying to maintain
prekid standards long after the children have arrived, you may be
dealing with one of the toughest family fragmentors: perfectionism. Feeling compelled to manage the perfect house, kids and career robs a parent of the ability to make choices and can drive anxiety levels off the charts. Encourage parents to discover the priorities
that drive them: Say, "Ask yourself, who am I trying to please?" and
"What do I really want?"

After posing these questions to herself, Andrea realized that, although cleanliness was next to godliness in her mother's home 30
years ago, she didn't much feel like wrestling her 3-year-old daughter, Meredith, into the bathtub every night. She decided to bathe

Meredith every other evening, and the less rigid schedule transformed bath time into a more pleasant experience.

4. Push parents to delegate responsibility. Many mothers, especially, say that it's easier to do everything themselves than to accept a less-than-perfect job by a spouse or hear kids complain that Mom is no longer "on call." Remind mothers, though, that pulling back may be tough on nerves in the short run but, as family members develop greater skill, they'll feel far less overwhelmed and resentful.

The most stressful chores that partners ought to share include getting kids ready in the morning, being responsible for dinner, and—most important—bedtime rituals. Chores can be delegated to children as early as age 3 or 4. These include helping to set and clean the table, sorting and folding laundry, watering plants, and caring for pets—in fact, any job that developmental skill and safety permit.

5. Address weekend mania. Weekends used to be a time to rest, but lately, many families are running themselves into the ground. Why? The modern emphasis on "quality time" has been misinterpreted to mean making sure kids are stimulated at all costs. This can mean weekends spent running from team sports to theme parks to movies. And any time not devoted to entertaining kids is consumed by those endless errands we don't accomplish during the week.

Scale down plans. Agreeing to every activity that kids or conscience demands builds up stress. Instead, encourage parents to plan events that better suit their specific situation and energy level. For example, Shelly, who has 4-year-old twins and a 7-year-old recently decided on a limit of one event per day: "Getting the kids ready for an activity requires so much preparation—clothes, snacks, drinks—that I decided to draw the line. My friends laugh at me, but that's all I can handle right now."

Suggest multipurpose errands that get the weekend chores done while parents can also fulfill more personal needs. For example, while shopping for the week's groceries, Lynette leaves her 2-year-old son at home with her spouse so she can meet friends for a quick cup of coffee. She also takes her current novel along to read on checkout lines. Adding in pockets of "self-time" helps Lynette feel less harried as she takes care of mundane but necessary tasks.

Remind clients to take a day of rest: Observe Saturday or Sunday as a family-centered day with no TV or outside activities. This may not be easy to arrange, since partners don't always see eye to eye on such matters and kids often put up a fuss because "it's boring." However, the struggle is worth it. "My partner and I work in high-pressure jobs, and 'family day' helps us keep home and work separate," says Jane. "The kids don't act up as much, knowing that they can count on our undivided attention."

Staying Connected during the Day

In fragmented modern family life, parents and kids often go for periods of time completely out of touch with each other. We cannot underestimate how different this is from previous eras: before technology, the economy focused on farming and manufacturing, small family businesses, and company towns. For better or worse, these enterprises kept family members highly interdependent. Kids not only saw their parents working up close but often participated in daily activities that centered on making a living. Obviously, the economy has changed. The more it becomes focused on delivering services, more of the kids I meet are completely uninvolved and even ignorant about what their parents do. This lack of concrete connection along with increased work and commuting hours makes it understandable that the number one complaint of children in my surveys is that "My parents are so busy, we don't have any time when they finally get home."

This daily disconnection is a serious issue—children and parents can end up feeling like ships passing each other in the night. Professionals need to address this with ways to stay connected during the day. Here are some:

1. Encourage parents to get kids "thinking of you" presents. It sounds simplistic but, according to the kids I've interviewed, this can make an enormous difference. It's not the expense that matters. In fact, these should be inexpensive gifts. It's a way of saying to a child, "You know what? During the day, while I was gone, I was thinking of you." I cannot overemphasize what a profound impact this makes. These are gifts to help kids stay connected during a difficult transition, not as a regular practice, Parents need to be told, "You know your child." Only do this when you know you're not giving a gift out of guilt.

2. Remind parents to write notes. Leave them around the house, for example, on the children's beds, after they've left for the day. With older kids, leave around a newspaper or magazine article of interest, something that can be casually strewn in areas they frequent. Crucial to such note leaving is this: tell parents *not* to ask a child, "Did you read the note? Did you like it?" This puts kids on the spot and takes away from the thought.

Leave notes in unexpected and creative places. Many mothers in my interviews told me about "I love you" notes they secretly include in lunch boxes. Use your imagination to help harried parents. A father I know put "Hi!" stickers on the TV screen. With teens, the mirror is a sure way for something to be noticed. E-mail is increasingly the communication of choice for many harried parents. Adolescents and even preteens love getting mail—and this is a nonintrusive way to reach out.

3. Call before coming home. Many of the well-functioning couples that we interviewed call home before they leave work. This allows them to find out what's happening around the house, rather than walking headlong into mayhem. It also gives kids a chance to tell Mom or Dad about problems at school, fights with sibs, or whatever concerns may be uppermost in their minds. Parents who phone home need less of a "transition time," for they have already begun to process the emotional environment they're about to enter.

Teach the Art of Parallel Communication

Many adults don't know how to talk to children. Either we're are too busy or we've been encouraged by an overly zealous mental health field to pounce on every tidbit a child throws our way. For stressed parents who overvalue communication opportunities, the research has some bad news. Kids open up *not* when we want them to, or on schedule, but in the middle of doing other things: in the car, on the bus, walking together, and playing games. For example, a child named Richie was acting out in school. It was a complicated situation. But all the therapeutic pyrotechnics in the world couldn't top this—mother and son took the bus to the clinic once a week. While sitting next to Mom, Richie gradually began to tell her things he'd never shared before. This was where the real connection between the two began to happen, and Richie's behavioral troubles started to lessen. This parallel communication is a piece of advice that helps parents and kids relate better around the house. For other techniques that increase expressiveness follow these guidelines:

1. Do not pounce. Many parents think, "If I don't answer now, my child will never want to talk to me again." So we pounce. And yet, children tell me this sends the wrong message. Ten-year-old Eddie put it so well when he observed, "I can't stand it when talking means more to my mom than it does to me. It makes me want to clam up." Get parents (and it's not bad advice for our own work) to cut down on our earnest eager-beaver reactions. Take your time—kids will feel less pressured and be more open.

2. Ask action-oriented questions. Mental health professionals and many modern parents love to ask silly questions like "How does that make you feel?" or they make quasi-therapeutic comments like "That must have made you very angry." In truth, this sort of thing drives many kids crazy. You need to ask *action* questions such as "*Who* was there?" or "*What* did they say?" or "*Where* were you?" or "*What* did you do then?" These are the questions that will get a child to tell the details of a story. Stay away from "why" and "when." Most kids (like most adults) have no idea *why* they do what they do; and the time concepts necessary for *when* questions are difficult for many children to conceptualize.

3. Be specific. One of the reasons kids give vague responses like "Fine" or "Nothing" when we ask, "How was school today?"

is, as children themselves have told me, "Well, they're not being specific enough. I can't remember." As mentioned before, during a workshop I ran, a very articulate child said to a group of stunned parents, "If my dad really cared, he'd know the details of what's going on." The most effective questions, then, are specific: "What happened with Vivian in math class today?" These jog kids' memories and show that we were involved and really listened to the details last time around.

4. Talk about *your* day. Speech pathologists have told me that most parents ask kids far too many questions. Think about what it's like for you to be asked one query after another. It really turns kids off; they feel poked, prodded, and in the spotlight's glare. So, the number of questions needs to be modulated, and statements should be interspersed about what happened to us adults during the course of a day. These invariably trigger kids' responses and improve their recall of the day's events.

For example, Sally found it amazing that each time she brought up a problem with her boss her normally reticent son, Alan, would chime in about some conflict he'd had that day with a friend or teacher. This phenomenon is so predictable that my wife and I regularly discuss specific events that have come up for ourselves, only to be drowned out by the stories these seem to trigger in our children. Dinner time is no longer a one-sided interview about our kids' lives.

5. Learn the art of indirect communication. Communication that is not always aimed right at the children is, paradoxically, far more interesting to them. Thousands of parents have vigorously agreed that as soon as two adults start speaking together or a parent picks up the phone, most kids feel compelled to butt in. If you really want a child to get involved, tell parents to *whisper* to each other. As soon as my wife, Stacey, and I would start to whisper to each other, we'd find our daughter, Leah, standing within 5 feet of us, looking at some wall as if she was inspecting the paint job. "There was nothing to look at," Leah admitted years later. She simply wanted to hear what we were saying—because, after all, we must have been talking about *her*!

Encouraging Parents to Get Interested in Kids' Interests

Mutual interests are crucial for today's disconnected families. For instance, a mother named Gigi came to me for advice about how to get closer to her young adolescent son, Aaron. "What's the boy interested in?" I asked. "He loves baseball, and he likes to read the statistics on Sunday." So I asked Gigi to spend 15 minutes (I'd first suggested every other day—we struggled together to find the just-tolerable level of change and arrived at 15 minutes once a week.), sitting with her son so she could learn a little about the world of baseball statistics. Gradually Mom started to hear that Aaron loved all the players who had some kind of physical injury and were underachievers. Guess what? Gigi finally "got" that Aaron, also an underachiever, felt much worse about his diagnosed reading difficulty than she'd ever realized. Mom never really understood this until she took an active interest in Aaron's passion and through it learned what was on his mind.

Another example: When I worked in Brooklyn, a child, James, came to our clinic. He had no interests and was so verbally mute that many teachers considered him retarded. It turned out that James's development was not delayed; it's just that none of the adults talked his language—cars! By discussing the car world with him, I found out who his friends were, who was "in" and who was "out." I encouraged his mother to do the same. Soon he asked her to go to a Monster Truck show, a real test of her commitment to greater connection. But despite her ears nearly exploding from the squeal of racing tires and engines, Mom felt plugged in *and* James began to talk to her about other matters. James started to make some progress in his life—better grades, less arguing around the house. Increasingly, he and his mom felt much more connected and cooperative toward each other.

What about interests that are almost repulsive to a parent: video games, rap music, and so on? These, too, are avenues of connection. For example, I said to one parent, Marie, "Go to one of those violent R-rated movies with your daughter. She's seeing them anyway." Mom agreed, and the girl reluctantly "allowed" Mom to accompany her (preventing adolescent shame by making Mom sit one row behind). This breakthrough of sorts got them talking though. It spread to many discussions about other culture crazes: fashion, sex, the hot new "hunks," and so on. To her own surprise, Mom got used to her daughter's interests, and while their tastes differed significantly, at least they weren't engaged in a hostile cold war with each other.

Encouraging Delay of Gratification

Modern culture is moving in just the opposite direction, and our growing need for instant gratification has several subtle yet profound consequences for connectedness in family life. Impatience and adversarial relationships permeate many homes saturated with pop culture. We don't realize how pervasive this is. Certain catchphrases ("Do it." "Just *do* it!" "Obey your thirst." "Do it *now!*") create an expectation in kids that they must be instantly gratified. Computer games, e-mail, and videos also reinforce instant gratification. They are so self-regulated, the activities are almost masturbatory, allowing kids to control the amount of frustration and impatience they can tolerate. But in life—school, friends, sports—this kind of self-regulation is impossible. Easily frustrated children often give up and withdraw, especially from difficult family relationships. How can you help parents and kids with this?

1. **Limit the amount of TV and video time.** Reducing TV and video time can feel overwhelming. Parents need to start small. Keep in mind that children (and many adults) are truly addicted to their electronic soul mates. For example, if a child watches 5 hours of TV a day, help a parent to cut it down to 4. This may not seem like a big change, but it engenders the idea that delay of gratification is necessary—and it begins the process of change.

The same limits apply to grade schoolers and adolescents who go on the Internet. From my discussions with kids and parents, I am beginning to find that junior e-mail easily turns into casual aggression. Since kids don't see each other's reactions, anything aggressive is relatively easy to say. And, for all it's wonders, the Internet also causes family diffusion. Any parent of a modern pre-teen or adolescent knows that kids are drawn to talk to so many people (at once) outside the home that the family at home practically disappears. Most parents report greater family connection when they limit Internet access to approximately a half hour a night.

Video games *must* be limited precisely because they reinforce instant gratification in a powerful way. Studies are beginning to show that simultaneous levels of stimulation—interaction, self-reg-ulation, and positive reinforcement—make video games one of the most effective means of learning (Steve Dorman, "Video and Com-puter Games: Effect on Children and Implications for Health Edu-cation," *Journal of School Health*, 67, 4, 1997). Unfortunately, the vast majority of games that kids choose are in the domain of fantasy and violence (both boys *and* girls), rather than educational.

That video games are a "gateway" toward aggression is increas-ingly known through the anecdotal reports of parents; they regu-larly complain of more sibling and play date fighting as soon as the "64" or play station is activated. There is no way around it—the amount of time that kids are allowed to play these games needs to be limited.

2. Put off private TV sets. Shockingly, across all socioeco-nomic levels in the United States, a majority of kids now have TV sets in their own rooms! Obviously, this has profound conse-quences on connections between family members. Use of separate TV sets cuts down on time spent with others. It also makes it im-possible for parents to share with their kids what they are viewing and doing. From hundreds of interviews and workshops, I've heard a clear message: put off private TV sets in the kids' rooms for as long as possible.

3. Monitor, monitor, monitor. The most powerful way to stay in charge as well as increase family connection is to monitor and remain deeply involved in kids' electronic activities. For exam-ple, Mike, who felt quite estranged from Delores, his budding young adolescent daughter, found little in common to talk about with her. When, with my suggestion, he began to watch one of her teenage soap operas, *Dawson's Creek*, the two instantly started to have more conversations. These times together also provided Mike with some understanding of the show's allure. Instead of reflexively prejudging and condemning it, Dad actually liked the program. Thus began a weekly ritual during which the two watched the show, scarfing down popcorn and having animated discussions about the characters' lives. Pretty soon no one called their house between 8:00 and 9:00 on Wednesday nights—father and daughter were engaged in a valued activity *together.*

Helping Kids Connect with Their Sibs

The quality of connection between siblings is often a real problem. But it is also an *opportunity* to create less family disconnection. Most parents think it's normal for there to be a lot of sibling friction, and we tend to overlook the negative consequences of this kind of aggression. While some sibling stress is inevitable, chronic hostility needs to be addressed. According to the families I've interviewed, when it comes to everyday stress levels, almost nothing else affects family life as much. Here's what you can do to help parents bring down the level of sibling tension:

1. A house divided cannot stand. Often, when a second child is born, new alliances are created: Dad pairs off with the older child as Mom tends to the infant. Over time, each parent gets to be more of an expert with one of the children. Eventually, the family divides right down the middle. You need to help change that. The simplest way is by encouraging families to do activities in different combinations. Initially, it may be very hard to get kids and parents past this natural "buddy" system, but it is dramatically effective.

For example, older brother Ryan was torturing "Daddy's favorite," Chris. I asked Dad to turn things upside down and spend a little extra time with Ryan. Dad decided to enter Mom's territory and convinced Ryan to go clothes shopping together. At first, Ryan was uncomfortable doing this "Mom activity" with Dad. But several afternoons of partner switching like this allowed Dad to become more an expert about Ryan. He learned whom he wanted to be like, who was on the fringe of the peer group, who was the coolest dresser, and so on. As the natural division in this house decreased, the amount of fighting between Ryan and Chris significantly lessened.

In another family, one of the boys was very rough with his younger brother. Mom was continually mad at the aggressive child. She tended to spend more time with the "victim" and be more affectionate toward him. This only increased the older sib's resentment. I asked Mom to spend some extra time learning one of the older child's favorite computer games. After a few weeks, this extra bit of attention made Mom and the older child feel closer; not surprisingly, some of the boy's hostility toward his brother decreased.

2. Address the sibling dance. There's often a dance between siblings in which one becomes labeled as the "perpetrator" and the other as the "victim." Subtly, though, the victim provokes the perpetrator, who is always blamed as the troublemaker. The victim can provoke an uproar in the most subtle ways, knowing exactly what drives her sib crazy: "He breathed on me," "She's making that disgusting face again," or "He crossed over his side of the line in the car." Understanding this dance lessens complaints about unfairness and breaks down static labels that quickly get assigned to each child. This is particularly important because labels tend to stick over time and become self-fulfilling prophesies: the angel becomes "perfect"; the devil becomes a "monster."

For example, Ethan had been labeled the "angel," while his mischievous elder brother Eddie was labeled the "troublemaker." For years, Eddie had complained that *perfect* little Ethan was the instigator of many battles and that his parents only saw the moments when Ethan retaliated. His mom and dad, not recognizing the sibling dance, kept attributing the trouble to Eddie. Over time, Eddie became an inveterate mischief-maker in school, living up to his label so well he was about to be thrown out. With my encouragement, the parents began to notice how Ethan instigated at least half of the fights. Behind their backs, he was subtly mocking, made faces and gurgling noises. After the parents were armed with this knowledge, Eddie began to be viewed more favorably, especially as Ethan became the focus of discipline. Change continued—Eddie behaved less abrasively around the house, and his parents started to offer him genuine attention and affection. Within a number of weeks, Eddie had significantly calmed down in school. Connections around the house were much more equal and everyone (even Ethan, who felt relieved at not having to be so perfect) was happier.

3. Find the special skills in each child. Help parents find the skill in each child that can be nurtured. The idea of treating siblings as if they were equal has never been proven to work. In fact, research shows just the opposite—it leads to greater self-comparison and friction. Instead, work on developing each child's uniqueness. Christine and Grace were two such children. Only 1½ years separated them, making it quite likely that they would be involved in competitive struggles. However, their parents were determined to find what was unique in each child. Over the years, I saw the wonderful results of their efforts. Christine became a superb soccer player. Her leadership and dedication to the team helped her develop better work habits in school. On the other hand, Grace had been an avid reader since she was a very young child. Though she, too, played soccer, at a certain point her mom and mom's partner did not push the game. Instead, they helped her focus on her love of learning. Grace values herself as an excellent student and, though not as serious about soccer, still likes to play. Because they are defined as unique individuals, the two girls fight less and are much closer sibs than one sees in many other families.

4. Insults are not inevitable. One of the biggest problems between siblings is that we think it is natural that they put each other down. Over time, many supposedly harmless insults become part of a child's self-definition. Obviously we can't, nor should we, stop all verbal roughhousing. Yet, we must find the insults that are truly toxic and lead to alienation between siblings.

Encourage parents to ask each child, "What are the two or three things your brother/sister says that bother you the most? That's what we're going to work on. The rest, you'll ignore." In one family, Eva requested that her two boys, Abe and Ned, list what each felt were the most hurtful put-downs. Abe chose "sissy"; Ned said "dumb" was the worst. Eva came up with a contract that each boy signed, promising not to use the specific insult or suffer serious consequences. Of course, Abe and Ned did not totally stop insulting each other, but finding the words that hurt the most definitely softened some of the rampant aggression around the house. Months later, Eva reported to me that this improvement had continued.

5. Intervene less. Research is beginning to show exactly what I've heard many times from veteran parents: the more adults get involved, the more kids seem to act up. Recently a woman who had 22 children was interviewed on this subject. She said the secret to the kids turning out OK (and to her own survival) was that she stopped getting mixed up in every spat, trying to be a fair judge. Unfortunately, she admitted to learning the secret late—after her *eighth* child. But this wisdom, born of hard work and tough experience, can help parents learn faster. Here's the key concept: tell parents to gradually cut down on interventions; they should intervene only when there's danger of physical harm. In every other situation, they should give kids a chance to work it out themselves.

This is not always easy for overprotective mothers or rigid fathers. For example, Diane, who had two young grade school girls, found it difficult to stay out of their squabbles. So, we worked on setting a just-tolerable change for her. In Diane's case, this meant keeping out of the middle only when (1) there were no people to be embarrassed in front of and (2) when they had no appointment they needed to get to. To her surprise, Diane discovered that if she stayed out of it when her girls argued over the rules of a game, or playing house, or any other minor disagreement, the results were nothing short of phenomenal. They almost always came up with compromises that were far better than the ones she'd previously tried to enforce.

Encouraging Everyday Rituals

During the interviews I conducted with school-age children, their number one request was for daily rituals. Child after child mentioned the importance of ordinary activities most adults take for granted: reading stories together, Friday night pizza while watching videos, a bedtime kiss every night. These ordinary rituals are anchors in the chaotic, frazzled world we live in. Infancy research shows that predictability is important even in the first weeks of life; this need only increases as families try to survive the pressure-cooker pace and logistical nightmare we call daily living. Besides being anchors in a chaotic world, rituals provide a time and reason to reconnect with each other. As one mom put it so poignantly, "If we didn't have Sunday night dinners together, I don't think I'd see my three adolescent kids at all."

1. Encourage what already works. Ask parents to write down a list of rituals they already do (an example of such a list is given in the accompanying box). Look for those ordinary routines that usually are taken for granted. For example, a fellow I grew up with ended up moving five times around the country with his family because of his teaching career. After discussing their daily routines, he and his wife both described a wonderful ritual previously taken for granted. Every night after dinner they would take a 10-minute walk around the block. The two came to see that this tiny ritual helped hold their family together through many dislocations.

2. Create intergenerational events. We live in a culture that glorifies youth and caters to youngsters so much that, inadvertently, the generations are often separated. For example, we begin with theme parties geared solely to the kids. These days, performers on the circuit are paid considerable fees to amuse children, leaving grown-ups on the sideline. We take children to play centers which didn't even exist two decades ago. Kid-centered restaurants, parks, and malls may be great in terms of stimulating our children but can be another wedge between the increasingly disparate worlds of parents and children. Family restaurants like McDonald's and Burger

A List of Family Rituals

No ritual is too simple or unassuming to be overlooked:

1. Bedtime routine
2. Reading together
3. Watching a favorite TV program
4. Cooking together or ordering in fast food
5. Downtime—doing "nothing" together
6. Helping mom or dad on a project
7. Religious services

King have added brilliantly designed, kid-activity areas. On the one hand, this is terrific—we can eat in peace while our kids play safely near by, on the other hand, together-time is further diluted. Because all these practices can make parents and children veritable strangers to each other, we need to create more intergenerational events. Get-togethers that include guests of all ages build kids' tolerance of older folks *and* non-child-focused activities.

For example, a family I know whose members are scattered within a couple of hours of each other have a weekly get-together held on Sundays. This is a time when kids and adults just hang out with each other. I've been struck by how comfortable these children are when conversing with grown-ups. Encourage parents to not panic when kids express the "B" word—boredom—which often terrorizes adults and convinces them to back away from intergenerational activities. As always, start small. Once a month may be fine at first. Over time, children learn, as I indicated above, to actually converse with adults and develop some ability to survive a few hours without an entertainment center.

3. Teach one's heritage. Children are steeped in the "second family" notion that "all that really matters is what's happening now!" Judging from the kids I meet and surveys conducted, youngsters don't know a lot about general history and, specifically, their own family's past. This historical ignorance adds to a disconnection in family life. Therefore, in order to ensure that children view adults as three-dimensional human beings who have feelings and experiences that predate the kids, it is vital to teach children their heritage.

Encourage parents to initiate stories about family history. Irene and Katherine, a couple I know, would often tell their children tales of their family's many emigrations from one country to the other during and after World War II. At first, the kids resisted these excursions into the past, but over time they began to see their parents and some of their distant relatives to be the heroes they really were. In another family, the parents used photographs, memorabilia, and old 16-millimeter movies converted to videos to make their history come alive. Again, what started out with whining on the kids' parts ended up in rapt attention, sitting on Mom's and Dad's laps.

All children should begin to know, starting by the time they're 3 years old, where they come from. Even adolescents can be lured into paying attention—if you follow a particular format: "I know this has *nothing to do with you*, and you're going to think *it's stupid*, but, when I was young . . . " Keep it very short—remember, attention spans are now measured in nanoseconds. Persist, because stories about one's heritage connect children to their roots, an avenue toward greater family connection.

Encouraging Spirituality

Anything that is bigger than children themselves creates connection within families. Eminent researchers like Robert Coles believe that even our youngest children want to know about God and heaven; they want to know what happens after life. In short, they need to know that there is something bigger than them. If you don't believe in God, then a philosophy or a cause may teach a message far more connected than "I'm number one."

Yet, we professionals, not always trained in the spiritual aspects of life, tend to overlook this. I was once consulting behind a one-way mirror with a family in which the mother left the house unattended, leading to a fire that nearly killed everybody. The group of counselors couldn't get anywhere with his mother. The reason we were stalled was that no one asked Mom, who was a devout Roman Catholic, whether she had made peace with what she had done. In fact, Mom believed she would go to hell because it was *her* responsibility that this fire had started. We belatedly included a priest in on the counseling and finally got Mom moving in her life.

Most times, fortunately, it shouldn't take such a horrible circumstance for professionals to recognize how important spirituality, in whatever form, is to family life. Be aware of this need, and help parents create more spiritual connection using the following strategies:

1. Engage in altruistic activities. Children gain an appreciation of themselves and their power to help by *doing*. Whether they wrap Christmas gifts in their church or help out in a soup kitchen or community center, doing good deeds encourages more positive feelings long after the activity itself. A striking example of this is a group called the Kids Care Club. This national organization grew out of an original afternoon during which kids helped an elderly neighbor clean up her yard. The children felt so good about what they had done that they organized another activity which attracted many other neighborhood kids—helping paint the outside of a nearby home. More families wanted to get involved, and now, several years later, the Kids Care Club is a national network that encourages children to do good in order to feel more connected to themselves and their families. The lesson is clear: good deeds lead to greater connection.

2. Encourage parents to teach their beliefs. Because of democratic child-rearing philosophies, many parents think it oppressive to teach absolute beliefs about right and wrong. Yet, longitudinal studies are beginning to show that children who hear clear messages about their parents' belief systems engage in less risky adolescent behavior. It's not just right and wrong that parents need to teach either. Kids learn a vocabulary for expressing certain feelings they might not be exposed to in the world of the "second family"—words like "blessed," "sacred," and "compassionate," to name just a few. Words lead to actions, and kinder actions certainly create greater connection in family life.

3. Praise random acts of kindness. Many of the parents who come to us do so because of conflicts and fighting at home. Professionals often lose sight of a fact that researchers such as John Gottman (*Why Marriages Succeed or Fail*, Simon & Schuster, 1994) are now making poignantly clear: every act of kindness in a family is like emotional money in the bank. It provides immunity from the wear and tear of daily living, as well as the more destructive exchanges that inevitably occur. So, encourage mothers and fathers not to ignore the good moments when one of the children shares a toy with his sibling or a portion of his favorite dessert or is helpful around the house. One mother, Martha, whom I met at a workshop, e-mailed me several weeks later, saying that she had never realized how rigidly focused she was on pointing out the problems while letting the occasional warmer, more generous moments slip by. "Now," said Martha, "I notice them and tell the kids. I underline it with a hug or a pat on the shoulder. It sounds so simple, but the atmosphere around our house seems very different."

Spirituality is a kind of insurance: "The next time we worship, or participate in a cause together, or count our blessings, we're not going to fight." If families can break destructive cycles long enough to serve in a soup kitchen together, they can often move on from a battle which only moments before had seemed like the most important matter in the entire world. Spirituality helps bring family disagreements down to their appropriate size.

Helping Families *Not* Get Organized Around Symptoms

Finally, remember that parents contact helping professionals because their kids have *symptoms*. You will often learn that most of their connectedness is around the anxiety, frustration, and anger that goes along with the trouble. If a girl is anorexic, just about every interaction is around food. If a boy is acting out, most exchanges are about discipline. This is one reason it's so difficult to relieve kids of symptoms. Unless you create ways of connecting *before* addressing problems, there are usually no satisfying relationships to look forward to. The old psychological wisdom then proves to be true—"A bad relationship is better than none at all"— and people cling to symptoms as a way of staying connected. So, even as you begin to focus on the main issue, help parents develop ways to connect with kids that have *nothing* to do with symptoms, trouble, or stress.

For example, I worked with a father, Ed, who could not stop lecturing Tony, his adolescent son, or nagging him about schoolwork. All they did together was connect around study problems. If I had pushed Ed to entirely disengage from these ineffective behaviors, the two wouldn't have anything left. So, I suggested that dad walk to school with his son every other day. It seemed like such a small change, but this little way of staying involved became important to both father and son. They began having discussions that weren't just around the boy's symptom, making it much easier to directly address the destructive manner in which schoolwork had been handled.

*   *   *

Keep in mind that family members, even in these fragmented times, still need to feel connected, no matter how upset or distant they are with each other. Symptoms will not disappear if connections are further threatened. So, use all the suggestions in this chapter as potential ways to motivate family members. Understanding that a more satisfying connection may be possible helps parents and kids find the courage to try out new behaviors. And, in the end, they feel less like families living under siege.

chapter eleven

At the Millennium

Toward a New Paradigm
for Working with Children
and Parents

As we enter the 21st century, the world of children and teens is saturated with a new level of frightening violence. During the hundreds of discussions I've had with teachers, guidance counselors, camp owners, clergy, and the other responsible adults in a child's life, no message has been clearer. They are deeply worried about a shift in the degree of cruelty, aggression, and day-to-day intolerance children often display. Being on the front lines as you, the reader, are, I am sure these same concerns have recently plagued you. Therefore, no state-of-the-art guide could ignore the disturbing increase in dissatisfaction and destructive and self-destructive behavior among our children. It is a challenge for the millennium. Our kids by their outrageous behaviors are *demanding* a reevaluation of how we conceptualize their experience and our efforts to help. This chapter is just that—a comprehensive paradigm, integrating the many suggestions in this guide with a perspective that explains what is happening and prepares us for what we need to do in the 21st century. Unlike the previous ones, this chapter is not so much about new *technique* as about a new perspective, a paradigm in progress. The techniques covered in Chapters 1–10 continue to be the most effective ways of dealing with kids and families; however, as you implement them it is critical that you understand how much kids' and parents' relationships are changing.

Professionals need to realize that the very definition of appropriate behavior is undergoing a significant, even frightening redefinition. We see this in our day-to-day work with children and families. It is often shocking what adults have become used to hearing in the course of daily family and classroom discussions.

For example, Jessica has just been told by her mother to stop watching TV and clean up the table. "Not now," Jessica says, without bothering to look up. "No, Jessica, I mean this minute," her mother, Diane, says sharply. "Later," Jessica responds almost absentmindedly. Mom stiffens and threatens her with a consequence: "Stop it now or there won't be TV tonight." Finally, she's got her daughter's attention. Jessica looks her mother squarely in the face and says, "Fuck you, Mommy!" Jessica is 8 years old.

Kids and the New Anger

"Fuck you, Mommy." The exhilarating horror of this phrase! How many adults today can imagine the consequence had they thought, let alone said, such a thing? Over the last 10 years, however, as these exchanges are increasingly part of everyday family interaction, it has become apparent to me that a major shift about acceptable behavior is taking place in parent–child relationships throughout the country. After all, Jessica is not a neglected or abused child in thrall to gang culture. Her parents are, in fact, middle-class professionals living in a comfortable suburb. Nor is Jessica "maladjusted" psychologically; she knows her parents love her, she earns good marks in school, and basically gets along well with other children. What is really shocking is that exchanges like this are so ordinary, they are a part of daily family discourse in America.

A father informs me that his 8-year-old son, when asked for the fourth time to turn off the computer game and straighten his room, snarls "Leave me alone, butthead!" A 10-year-old girl, told by her mother to finish her homework, barely glances up, utters under her breath, "What an asshole," and continues to play. I hear the "flailing tantrum" story over and over: a parent directs a child not to chew gum or to stop playing and get ready for bed; the child responds by hurling himself at the parent, flailing away with small fists at the adult's face and chest in a frenzy of anger. One therapist told me that a girl he had been seeing expressed her jealousy of an unborn sibling not by the usual array of anticipatory anxieties but by smashing a baseball bat into her mother's pregnancy-swollen belly.

After the series of tragedies our country has gone through in terms of schoolyard killings, we are no longer entirely surprised by news of gun-wielding preteens murderously venting fury on classmates and teachers. But we are still not remotely prepared to see intense (if, so far, less lethal) anger in kids 5, 6, and 7 years old. And yet, in 150 interviews with an economically, socially, and ethnically diverse group of young children I conducted *a year before* the Littleton shootings, I was startled to hear about the casual explosiveness in young kids whose parents obviously cared about them. "A few times a week, I get so mad, I go into my room and just rip it apart," I was told over and over by angel-faced innocents as they sat in the classroom. "I beat up on my brother and sister whenever I get mad," reported numerous open-faced youngsters. "When I get really, *really* angry," one 7-year-old girl lisped, summarizing what dozens of other children had expressed, "I go into the bathroom, shut the door, and scream as loud as I can!"

It is not just parents who are feeling the brunt of the explosive defiance that seems to be spreading like a virus through the ranks of America's children. Recently, I attended a Little League softball game led by an experienced coach, and watched it turn into a free-for-all: one 7-year-old, enraged after he struck out, grabbed home plate and ran off in a howling tantrum; another child, tagged "out," physically attacked the boy who had tagged him; a kindergartner, when she was called out by the umpire, ran up to him, screamed, "I hate you" and actually kicked him hard three times in the shins. All this in a friendly neighborhood game for kids and their families.

In interviews with important nonparental adults in kids' lives—

teachers, coaches, principals, community leaders, camp owners—I heard about the same disturbing pattern of anger and even disdain for adults, manifested not by hulking high school wrestlers but sometimes by the tiniest of tykes under 4 feet tall. One eminent children's theater director says that in 25 years of producing plays he has seen an increasing disrespect for him and his colleagues by his young charges: "I can't describe the enormity of change in the way children behave. I can no longer count on having their respect and attention merely because I am the adult and a teacher. Now half the struggle is just to get them to begin to listen to my directions." Even therapists are taken aback by breathtakingly raw affronts to adult authorities. Expert clinicians have told me that it is not at all unusual for grade- or middle-schoolers to look them dead in the eye, say "Who do you think *you* are?"—then get up and march out of the session.

Surveying this ravaged terrain, one cannot help but wonder why kids are this angry. What is going on that is so wrong between parents and children, often making it seem as though we are walking on a field of delayed-action high-explosive land mines? In large part, it's because, like deer frozen in the headlights of an oncoming car, parents at all ends of the political and economic spectrum are often utterly at a loss about how to provide leadership in their own families.

Parents and the New Anger

Parental Confusion

What do fathers and mothers do these days when their young child curses at them or goes into flailing tantrum mode or daily beats up a younger sibling? Not very much, as it turns out. Speaking for many, Melanie described her reaction when 6-year-old son, Eric, hit her and screamed at her in the supermarket: "I didn't know whether it was better to smack him on the spot or let him get his feelings off of his chest so they wouldn't fester." Other parents respond with intense rage and unenforceable punishments. In the face of her daughter's "fuck you," Jessica's mom immediately spanked her and threatened, unconvincingly, to take all TV away for a whole year. Several weeks later, while they were watching TV together, another version of the same incident occurred.

With the constant shifts in child-rearing approaches, parents have become so anxious not to do the *wrong* thing that they often become paralyzed. For example, 10-year-old Mindy had been invited to a party that night where she said the kids would be playing make-out games. "What should I do," Mindy asked her mother, Ann, "when they start kissing?" But Ann was as unsure as her little girl. Finally, after what seemed like an endless hesitation, she offered, "In the end, it's whatever makes *you* feel comfortable with who you are," a wishy-washy, unsatisfying answer that left Ann discouraged and Mindy very annoyed. Later, Ann confided to me that she truly doesn't know what would be better, letting the child "harmlessly" explore her emerging sexuality or setting strict limits that she might rebel against—and choose not to confide in her next time.

Bill, the father of depressed 13-year-old Jason, was in an equally serious quandary. After a couple of lonely years without friends, Jason had finally seemed to find a buddy—a classmate he brought home during lunch period. The tentative friendship seemed a real breakthrough except for one tiny detail: the two boys spent the lunch hour in Jason's room smoking dope. Should Bill ignore the massive infraction of school discipline, not to mention state and federal drug laws, in relief and exhilaration that his son had found a new chum, or should he crack down on illegal and dangerous behavior? Which was worse for the boy—being a friendless and possibly scapegoated loner in school or a budding pothead with a pal?

Moral Relativism

Adults are not only confused by their child's anger, they often seem to have lost their own moral direction. What, for example, happened to Chrissie, who screamed at the umpire and kicked him in the shins at the Little League game? Incredibly, her mother, who was watching, did not reprimand her; the umpire did not kick her out of the game; and a few minutes later, Chrissie got the weekly achievement certificate she'd "earned"—a red ribbon for her participation.

Moral relativism also seems to have become the collective attitude of what I call, in Chapter 7, the "second family"—the kiddie culture of peers and media that is often more important, and more visible, to children than the "first families" of their parents and siblings. Although young children I have interviewed—5, 6, and 7 years old—strongly believe in right and wrong and are angry when their parents fail to set rules, by fourth or fifth grade they begin talking in ominously relativistic terms about moral issues. Much to the dismay of adults, many children, responding to the Columbine murders, make remarks like, "I don't think what they did was right, but I don't completely blame them either. Those kids had their reasons—they were treated badly, and anybody can crack under certain conditions."

In 1996, the *Rockford Register Star*, an Illinois newspaper, gave us a glimpse into the second family's moral code. The newspaper polled hundreds of teens in heartland America, asking them what moral guidelines they followed. "There aren't any," these kids answered almost unanimously, "You only need to treat others the same way they treat you." Almost none of the teenagers, boys or girls, were prepared to label any behavior, no matter how noxious, simply right or wrong.

More disquieting, and perhaps more instructive, few of these kids had ever considered that adults might in some way be able to guide them in making decisions about issues of right or wrong. And why should they? Most of the grown-ups in their lives don't understand the details of second-family living or believe in their own ability to redirect their children—a failure kids pick up on only too well.

The Shifting Tides of Child-Rearing Advice

In truth, the cyclical waves of often contradictory advice thrown at parents over the past 30 years may be part of the confusion. As parents scramble to do what works, they try out the latest one-size-fits-all theory, only to find it superseded a little later by a new popular orthodoxy. Different parents get hooked on different child-rearing techniques, which tend to swing crazily back and forth between poles of permissiveness and toughness, regardless of whether these off-the-rack approaches are actually appropriate for *their* individual child. Eight-year-old Peter, for example, has gotten into another bruising battle with his little brother, who screamed in pain. Their mother, Hillary, tried an approach based on Thomas Gordon's Parent Effectiveness Training (PET) model (gaining popularity during the early 1970s) in reaction to strict Victorian child-training methods). PET emphasizes the importance of allowing children to express themselves freely and warns of psychological stultification if we suppress the child's inner spirit. Using "active listening" techniques, Hillary asked open-ended questions to help her sullen boy express and neutralize his feelings of jealousy. The more she used this kind of therapy-speak, the more tight lipped he became. "Oh, forget it," Peter finally said in disgust, and walked away.

The "tough love" approach, with its emphasis of setting limits and quashing what was now felt to be too *much* expressiveness, followed hard on PET, and that is where 12-year-old Jenny's parents decided to put their money. Jenny had been drinking, hooking up with lots of boys, staying out way past her curfew and doing poorly in school. Her father, Bob, already overly rigid, gave Jenny ironclad threats on bottom-line consequences, but hesitated enforcing them. Two days after his hell-and-brimstone sermon, Jenny didn't come home at all, having found a place to crash with some loosely supervised kids in the neighborhood.

As the knowledge of widespread family abuse and incest surfaced during the late 1970s and early 1980s, the pendulum in child-rearing advice swung back toward protecting and "empowering" children. Thus, the self-esteem movement was born, encouraging both parents and children to believe that every child was "special" just for "being a person." Part political, part reaction to inexorable increases in childhood disorders and acting out, the self-esteem surge was overtaken by an even bigger wave, emphasizing "family values." During this period, parents were exhorted that if they taught their kids morality, psychology would take care of itself.

During the early and mid-1990s, neurobiological discoveries caused the tides to shift once more in favor of the biological underpinnings of various childhood difficulties, now given labels like pervasive developmental disorder, attention-deficit disorder, or affective disorders. The role of parents and professionals became that of helping children take medication or compensate for problems that were largely beyond conscious control. Most recently, in reaction to this biological trend, regarded in some circles as a flimsy mechanism for providing alibis to spoiled and undisciplined kids, authoritarianism is making a comeback. "Children should be punished for every act of disobedience, no matter how small," intones John Rosemund, a main spokesman for the new movement. Spanking is highly recommended by conservative psychologist James Dobson. Currently, in the shadow of the school shootings, there is a legislative movement afoot to post the Ten Commandments in every schoolroom in America.

Kids and the New Anonymity

"Sometimes," says one of the fifth graders in my study, "I get the feeling my parents don't know me." "Mine too," yells an irate classmate from across the room. "We don't spend time together—we're always so busy in my house." Just about every child nods enthusiastically, some with obvious fury.

Do We Really Know Our Children?

It is logical that many parents buy great quantities of off-the-rack advice because, stretched to the limits as they are, they do not really know their kids. They cannot always tell the ways in which their kids are unique individuals because they just do not spend enough direct one-on-one time with them. The hard truth is that many parents may love their children but do not create the time to pay attention to them. They do not really hear them. They do not really see them.

This sounds harsh, and it is a bitter pill for overworked parents to swallow, particularly those who feel their lives are already intensely child centered. Indeed, there are recent indications that parents today spend the same, if not more, time with their families than June and Ward Cleaver ever did on "Leave It to Beaver." But when we examine what kind of time spent with one another we get a troubling picture of what so-called family togetherness actually looks like these days. Family members may be spending time *near* each other, in the same house, engaged in parallel but separate activities, and not remotely doing things together. Indeed, a long-distance phone conversation can provide a much closer and more intimate experience of connection than a typical evening in the bosom of the modern American family. Mother, for example, may be supervising her 5-year-old in the bath while calling work to arrange a meeting for the next day; sister is e-mailing several buddies and talking with yet another friend on the phone; Dad (if he lives at home, or if it's his weekend with the kids) is busy finishing up a report, looking up every 10 minutes or so to announce it's nearly bedtime to whatever child might actually be listening.

There is nothing inherently evil about any of this—it's normal family life in America—but it is no way to get to know your own family. Kids understand this. They are angry and yearn for what they are not getting. In my conversations with children from prekindergarten to sixth grade, the kids overwhelmingly indicated that what they wanted most from their parents was more time, as in *undivided* attention: "I want my mom to stop being so busy and just play with me." "I love when my dad sits next to me and we watch movies together." "Last week my mom and dad took me bowling, and it was great!" "I want my mommy to lie down with me every night." I don't believe this is simply more whining by a generation of spoiled kids. These are the heartfelt responses of children who are desperate to be *seen*, truly *known*, rather than scheduled or psychologized.

The "Second Family" as the New Parent

What happens to children when they do not get the kind of undivided personal attention they need from their parents—or when they lack confidence in the capacity of their parents to guide them? Where do they look to find something that promises to assuage their yearnings for attention? Nature abhors a vacuum, and for American children, the great roaring hurricane of the mass media culture—particularly the culture of celebrity—rushes in to fill the psychic void that the family used to fill.

Twenty years ago, I rarely heard about celebrity fantasies in my work with kids; now, I rarely don't. Increasingly, children answer my questions by stating that their greatest wish is to be near a celebrity.

This is sad, but it is less ominous than the hunger within many kids to achieve celebrity status themselves, as if this were the one best bet for achieving the attention and sense of being known that seems to elude them. For most of the kids I interviewed, the lesson of Littleton was the indubitable celebrity that the shootings conferred on the shooters. The Columbine High School killers were ultimately successful, said many of these children, because their acts made them famous. Perhaps in a celebrity-drenched culture, most of us occasionally want to be famous, but for children who are furious because they can't get the personal attention of the people they love and need the most, the desire to be seen can become an all-encompassing and toxic need. In a medium of fragmented families whose members live parallel lives, in which children often feel more catered to than truly known, where off-the-rack child-rearing techniques complicate more than they resolve and moral relativism is the norm, the culture of celebrity is a potentially inflammable ingredient.

Kids who commit publicly violent acts have found the metaphor that describes the pain of, as well as the solution for, their invisibility. They engage in such behavior precisely because it makes an unknown person instantly and uniquely recognizable. In such children's minds, violence appears to be the perfect antidote to the unaddressed anonymity of their lives.

What We Need to Do

What are we to do with a problem of such substantial dimensions? How can family counselors help parents get to know their children better, reclaim them from the casually violent mass culture, and raise them to become strong and moral adults? Our track record inspires little confidence. Most family professionals, myself included, are not only unprepared for the current crisis in child rearing, we actually mirror in our professional practice the same social and cultural phenomena that sap the good sense of parents. If mothers and fathers do not know their own children very well, as counselors we don't get to know them that much better. Counselors, and even overburdened teachers, regularly dismiss a child from meetings so that we can work with the real problem, presumably the parents. As professionals—counselors, teachers, clergy—we have little training in child development and almost no idea about how to talk to kids, one on one. Children, angry that their parents don't listen to them or know them, aren't likely to feel any better heard by us helping professionals.

And if kids are being raised in a climate of dangerous moral relativism, our carefully cultivated, value-free neutrality has made us *proud* to claim that we do not set standards of right and wrong either; the closest we come to standing by any particular principle is our unflinching belief in the notion of family hierarchy. But without a firm set of values for raising children, we can't be much help to parents floundering around in their own moral confusion.

Toward a Personal and Specific Approach

During the last decade, as I increasingly saw myself struggling with these issues, I painfully concluded that if the mental health profession were writing a book about child rearing, the pages would be just about empty. Despite our extensive training, we have simply not been prepared to help parents raise their kids in today's culture. So several years ago, in the throes of this growing professional crisis, I began a project of exploration and research with several questions in mind. Would it be possible to build a different kind of paradigm for raising children that would encompass each child's individuality, while providing some substantial insights about what all children need in an era of enormous confusion among parents? I aimed for a *personal* and *specific* approach to address the violence-festering anonymity many children feel, one that provided dependable guidelines for child rearing without becoming just another technique-driven manual for raising everychild.

In the course of this project, I combed the child-development literature of the past three decades, unearthing some relatively undiscovered gold mines of information. One such example was a longitudinal study published in the *Journal of the American Medical Association* in 1997 (Peter Bearman, Jo Jones, & Richard Udry, "A Longitudinal Study of Adolescent Health") on 14,000 economically and culturally diverse adolescents over several years. Another was the research of the Johnson Institute, one of the largest drug treatment and research facilities in the country, which followed almost 100,000 youngsters for a decade (Student View Survey, *High Risk Transitions*, 1993). I was not looking for the latest spectacular *New York Times* Science Section finding; rather, I wanted to discover what, if anything, has been *consistently* regarded by child researchers over the years as critical for raising emotionally healthy children.

I was stunned to discover the convergence among these sources. The scientific research shows categorically that every child is an idiosyncratic individual, not only different from other kids but from her own siblings. Over the last 5 years, research has demonstrated an enormous variation in neurological hardwiring, leading to a range of temperamental differences. It stands to reason, then, that any new child-rearing approach must recognize the child in all his individuality, and it must promote a good "fit" between a parent's approach and the child's own personality.

What this means is that it is virtually impossible for any prepackaged technique to be uniformly applied without creating in children even greater anger at not being seen. One robust self-willed boy may actually respond well to firm punishment, whereas for another a parent's raised voice may do the trick. For some children, like my own son, Sammy, yelling or even using a harsh tone reduces a child to tears and creates tremendous resentment. Some children thrive on continual praise offered directly and generously, whereas others avert their eyes and seem more annoyed than pleased. The latest research essentially corroborates these reactions:

all kids are very different from the get-go. They have what might be called a distinct and essential *core*—a constellation of emotional and intellectual attributes that vary dramatically from child to child, an "acorn" of a self, as psychologist James Hillman suggests, that struggles to be recognized—and leads to anger when it isn't.

Healthy Children Need to Develop Certain Key Attributes

Another even more resounding message emerged out of my review of both formal and informal data: children need certain fundamental attributes in order to develop a strong inner sense of themselves—core skills to maintain the core self. Developmental theory that has held sway since World War II is not necessarily correct: child skills do not always just "click in" at the appropriate age. Every child has core attributes that seem to come naturally, but other skills need nurture. Self-esteem, it turns out, is not a birthright. It cannot be built without internal substance to support it.

The skills or attributes needed by every child fell into four broad categories that are at particular risk these days. First, all the sources indicated that, despite our ambivalence toward adhering to any authority, children need to feel *respect* for their parents and other adults. Respectful kids have clear expectations of what is required of them by important adults in their lives and are willing to follow through on these requirements. The research clearly demonstrates that, far from feeling oppressed by the obligation to look up to their elders, respectful children feel more secure and less angry in their daily lives and are better able to resist being drawn into risky behavior by peers. Second, children need the capacity for *mood mastery*—especially in this frustration-averse culture. It is critical for parents to help kids learn to moderate their own internal emotional states, to know how to calm themselves down when upset or angry. Without such internal resilience kids turn to outside influences—most often the second family—for structure and soothing. Third, even very young children in day care centers, nurseries, and preschools must learn what I call *peer smarts*. This is not only the ability to make and keep friends, but the sense to know when to walk away from friendships that are harmful or demeaning. Finally, every child needs to develop communication skills that I refer to as *expressiveness*. This is *not* the sophisticated glibness that today's kids all seem to be skilled at, but the ability to talk about what really matters—to talk about feelings, friends, dreams, wishes, and frustrations. Without this "emotional literacy," as school consultant Michael Nerney calls it, children cannot help but express anger in endless and destructive ways.

From these basic four attributes, several other related skills have cropped up both in the research literature and repeatedly in my own work with children and parents, for a total of 10 core skills or attributes (see the accompanying box). Some, like *expressiveness*, seem obvious in the context of counseling and education. Others, like *focus* and *passion*, are not so obviously part of most child professionals' vocabulary. But teaching a child how to focus, for example, will help him not only pay attention in school and on the playing field, but give him the most important tool: enjoyment of learning. Engaging a child's *passion*—for a hobby or interest or school subject—will nurture her innate enthusiasm and protect her from the virus of the supercool ennui afflicting so many kids these days.

Other skills—*caution* and *gratitude*—sound almost reactionary in today's laissez-faire climate. Children, though, have never before had such a need for caution—an ability to stop, think, and weigh the impact of actions on themselves and others before being swept away into some metaphorical mosh pit of the kiddie culture. Related to respect is gratitude, which sounds perhaps the most antiquarian of all the skills but is one of the most important. Gratitude nurtures in a child both a realistic recognition of what adults have done on her behalf and possibly a budding sense of faith and spirituality.

I purposely labeled these skills to sound ordinary rather than psychological or diagnostic. They are words used on a daily basis that resonate more deeply than the distancing terminology we're used to. Kids and parents relate more to whether they can *focus* on a task than they do to the diagnosis of attention-deficit disorder; parents worry about whether their child is *cautious* rather than whether she will act out. The aim is to help clients feel personally known in

Ten Core Attributes of Children Who Thrive

These are the 10 attributes of a strong core self, along with suggestions for how therapists and parents can help strengthen in children of all ages those skills they believe are most at risk:

- **Mood mastery.** Model specific ways to soothe intense emotional states—anger, anxiety, fear—that fit a child's particular temperament.
- **Respect.** Be clear about expectations, and know how to follow through with reasonable consequences when they are not met.
- **Expressiveness.** Match communication to a child's particular preferences, including communicative style, most accessible time of day, and degree of directness that can be tolerated.
- **Passion.** Know the ways to encourage love of learning—praising appropriately, dealing with disappointment, competitiveness, and perfectionism.
- **Peer smarts.** Teach a child to trust his feelings about friends, to try active solutions to relationship problems, and to walk away when nothing works.
- **Focus.** Organize activities—amount, duration, and complexity—that allow kids to stick with tasks and to succeed.
- **Body comfort.** Help a child accept the way he looks—to think but not obsess about it, to avoid struggles around food, and to be aware of sexual attitudes that affect self-image.
- **Caution.** Be open and directive enough that children will seek guidance before first-time events and not be afraid to discuss difficulties afterward.
- **Team intelligence.** Teach kids the immutable laws of group dynamics so that they can function well with others without losing their individuality.
- **Gratitude.** Understand how to instill healthy appreciation and nurture the roots of spirituality.

our presence, creating a language of change that addresses the anonymity of family life and standard therapy practice.

Does every child have to become strong in every skill? No, but the glaring absence of one, say, *body comfort* or *respect*, can seriously compromise a child. On the other hand, strengthening even one core attribute begins the healing process. Developing respect for adults and what they have to say, for example, is likely to strengthen a child's sense of caution, his capacity for gratitude, and perhaps his ability to focus successfully on schoolwork. Are these the only core skills a child will ever need? Not necessarily, but these skills have been proven essential at this time, in this age, and especially in this culture. As the *Zeitgeist* changes, we will surely reevaluate current attributes or add new ones.

Nothing is written in stone. This is a paradigm in progress, a way of saying when it comes to child rearing and family therapy that we cannot be where our field was several decades ago, before we were conscious of the undeniable facts of gender, race, and class. We can no longer afford to confine ourselves to the airy vagueness of abstract family process and ignore the content of what parents should actually do. Therapeutic neutrality aside, we must stand for something. And, in this anonymous yet highly charged second-family world, it needs to be the strengthening of a child's core self. This entails knowing the sum and substance of healthy child development, bringing children into counseling to learn more about who they are, and offering informed feedback and guidelines to parents using our knowledge to help them fit better with their children.

We need to encourage parents to strengthen in their own children the core values and skills required to channel aggression into emerging responsibility.

The New Paradigm in Action

We've gone over many techniques to deal with parents and kids. Use the accompanying checklist to jog your memory. In reporting the following cases I assume your knowledge of them and do not repeat them in this chapter.

Summary Chart

1. Gathering information:
   - Enactments
   - Stories from home
   - Task assignments

2. Diagnosis: spot underlying difficulties and possible referrals.

3. Get kids to talk using various techniques described in Chapter 10.

4. Stay aware of your emotional reactions during meetings; they may be valuable signals of what to address.

5. Ask for the details about daily life; become acquainted with how much pressure the family feels:
   - Scheduling
   - Pace
   - Weekends versus weekdays

6. Find out who's in charge of the "endless list":
   - Who calls you
   - Who comes in
   - Who pays

7. Remember main points of handling "difficult parents":
   - Go slow
   - Be empathetic
   - Find just-tolerable anxiety

8. If you're dealing with an adolescent, keep in mind peers in her "second family" who may be important.

Finding Passion

Fourteen-year-old Jay was sent to me because of two outrageously public displays of anger. The first was inviting 300 of his closest friends to a parent-free suburban home, which was trashed by the raucous guests; several weeks later, Jay was caught with a couple of other boys vandalizing a county office building.

When I learned the details of Jay's day-to-day life, I did not remain neutral—I silently used the template described above, evaluating his core skills, trying to determine which are stronger, which weaker. After a few sessions, it was clear that Jay had no compelling interest. Glaringly, his core self had a numbing lack of *passion* for anything but second-family pursuits—his video games, his CDs, his friends.

We live in a time characterized by a tyranny of cool. But a passion for something other than the pop culture itself builds the kind of connections that are usually antidotes to aggression. A passion for music, art, science, horseback riding, whatever, requires kids to abide by certain rules and delay immediate gratification. Most often, it also engages the young person in a learning relationship with a responsible adult—a mentor, coach, or teacher. Finally, kids with passion tend to hang out with peers involved in the same or other interests, those who are not completely absorbed in second-family values.

I once would have explored Jay's feelings and asked him to talk about what led to his behavior. But now I had matters of content to take care of. I quickly discarded professional neutrality and told Jay straight out that he sounded bored most of the time, that *passion* was missing from his life. This was not presented as an open-ended question ("Do you ever feel your life lacks passion?") but as a direct, clearly stated guideline from an expert in child rearing. Jay responded with pro forma adolescent disdain: "Oh, yeah? What big interest did *you* have as a kid?" Jay grumbled about how stupid the very word "passion" was, that nobody he knows can stand a gung-ho dork—and the session was over.

Later that week, I told Jay's parents that they must help Jay develop a passion—one deeply engaging extracurricular activity. They were taken aback not to hear more off-the-rack advice that greater hierarchy and discipline were needed. The idea of passion didn't exactly make them happy either. Several weeks later, the three finally hammered out a deal that could only happen in postmodern America: Jay would be allowed to get some previously banned X-rated magazines in exchange for taking up an extracurricular activity.

Jay sulkily picked out a science project on ways to grow outdoor plants indoors (its potential illegalities were intriguing to the boy) and began working on it with another kid and their teacher. Within a few months, Jay and his science buddy became good friends—they did homework together and crammed for tests together. They also played quick hands of poker during free periods and occasionally drank to excess together. But as Jay's grades steadily rose from D's and C's to mostly B's, his disengaged flatness diminished.

Even more remarkable was the effect of Jay's connection with the project's adviser. This first nonremedial adult in Jay's life since fourth grade happened to have a zeal for learning and an openness to irreverent discussion, and Jay began to develop an embryonic ability to talk to other adults—including his mother and father. He actually asked his dad for help on the project, and every so often he even revealed day-to-day life events to his mother. As Jay spent more time with his study buddy and his rediscovered parents, his attention was drawn away from acting out. He started a study group, coauthored an ingenious (and completely legal) crib sheet for math tests, and asked out a girl he'd secretly been hot about for years. A year and a half later, his development is still on course. Jay is no longer a dead-eyed kid in thrall to the mass culture. He seems to have literally come home after a long voyage in an alien land.

Teaching Expressiveness

Most professionals are aware that today's kids, so glib about any and all subjects, are often totally unable to talk with parents about what really matters. The research clearly shows that a lack of *expressiveness* damages a child's ability to problem-solve and stay away from risky behavior. The reason, however, for poor expressiveness is not always a generic emotional muteness that strikes like a virus when children become preteens, but the failure of the adults in their lives to recognize the child's own particular *style* of expression. Just as counselors have tended to impose one particular mode of expressiveness onto children in sessions, parents in their well-meaning effort to communicate with their offspring may be speaking a language their particular child can't understand or even tolerate.

So it was with Eddie, a 13-year-old boy who came in with his father, Burt, following a divorce in which his sister and mother had moved to another part of the country. Burt, traumatized by the separation, was also deeply troubled by Eddie's being utterly disrespectful and uncommunicative to both him and his extended family. Though verbally almost mute, Eddie "spoke" in the way he appeared: he had a bright orange Mohawk hairstyle, prominent tattoos, multiple piercings in his ears and tongue, and showed up at staid family gatherings in gangsta' rap attire—hooded sweatshirts, huge baggy jeans, and brand name sneakers with untied laces. Sitting alone and sullen in the corner of the room, he answered the solicitations of his worried relatives with grunts and grimaces.

Several years ago, I would have attempted to provide a forum for father and son to open up together. Now, I was on a different, much more specific path: in order to promote verbal expressiveness which Eddie greatly needed, I wanted to learn about the boy's basic communicational style. So I asked Burt to describe to me Eddie's language development. Furthermore, I inquired into Burt's and his wife's own developmental histories. Interestingly, his wife had been shy, less likely to initiate conversation, and occasionally became tongue tied. Eddie's lack of verbal expressiveness was not simply depression or defiance—it was one measure of his unique personality, an inheritance from his mother that was exacerbated by his father's loquaciousness.

I told Burt I couldn't stop Eddie's nonverbal but outrageous public statements until the boy could acquire better core skills at expressing himself: "You have to change the way you talk to Eddie," I said bluntly. "You have to stop yelling, and you can't hammer him with questions. His system can't absorb it—you may not like it but this is the child you have." "How can I quiet down," Burt, the attorney, hollered back at me, "My whole family's been talking this way forever. I make my living talking like this."

Over several months of practice, Eddie's father became adept at giving his son time to respond to one question before firing off another and the atmosphere at home began subtly but unmistakably to change. As Eddie realized his father would listen quietly when *he, Eddie*, wanted to talk, and would respond more slowly and evenly, the content of the conversations grew more intimate. One evening, during a TV commercial, Eddie stunned his father by, for the first time, bringing up the divorce.

Burt, seeing these unexpected changes, told me about a deeper hurt—resentment that Eddie did not appreciate him, that he took his fatherly steadfastness entirely for granted. Eddie's chronic rudeness had left Burt feeling that nothing he had ever done for the boy counted for much.

Instilling Gratitude

In fact, Burt was right. *Gratitude* is a core attribute missing in many children today. According to a growing body of research, real gratitude, discouraged by a second-family culture that expects instant gratification, is one of the basic steps toward empathy. It slowly emerges from children's realistic awareness of their own dependency and the efforts most parents and teachers actually make on their behalf. Furthermore, gratitude helps kids feel small in a healthy way. They learn to recognize that they are not the center of the universe and are often dependent upon the good will of others.

I agreed with Burt that he had a right to expect gratitude from his son and said that he deserved and ought to expect some acts that demonstrated his son's grateful appreciation, such as going to family events with him. I suggested that, instead of ordering Eddie to attend family functions, he might say to him, "I really need you to do this. It is embarrassing and hurts me when you do not come." Getting ask-for-no-help Burt to say the word "need" required several family-of-origin sessions. When he finally looked Eddie in the eye and spoke to him quietly, Burt was amazed that his son did not stomp out of the room in a disdainful rage; true, Eddie sighed and rolled his eyes, but he also actually listened and nodded. Burt, slightly encouraged, took another chance. Again, instead of demanding that Eddie eat dinner at home, Burt said that he really needed the boy home once or twice a week—he felt lonely and sad eating dinner every night by himself. This approach, stressing Burt's vulnerability, dovetailed with Eddie's underlying sensitivity and exactly fit what Eddie needed. The two started having occasional meals together. Most of the time, they sat silently watching the tube, but every so often they found themselves having open conversation about what had happened during the day—ordinary conversation of good friends as well as father and son.

As *expressiveness* and *gratitude* slowly strengthened and he became more known to his father, Eddie's outrageous and provocative statements slowly disappeared from his neon-like body. Now, several years later, Eddie is successfully graduating high school, having been taken under the wing of a master martial arts teacher—an older man who, interestingly, speaks very slowly and demands a high degree of respectful attention and gratitude.

Strengthening Peer Smarts

Unlike Jay and Eddie, 12-year-old Alicia had *passion* and *expressiveness* to spare, and lavishly exhibited them as a committed actor. Smart, pretty, thin, and involved, she completely mystified her parents by her frequent tantrums and almost violent arguments with peers. Alicia publicly snapped at startled playmates. She was, at best, a diva with friends and a demon toward others. During several meetings I learned from Alicia that she had a rather striking absence of *peer* smarts. She continually seemed to say "yes" to the wrong kids, while alienating friendlier and more emotionally solid kids by being unpredictably mean: Zach, her 14-year-old heartthrob, said to her, "You're kind of ugly, but I like you anyway," and then kissed her. Befuddled by this mixed message, Alicia let him kiss her and felt hurt and confused for the rest of the day. Later on, a female classmate sensed Alicia's bad mood and approached her with a smile and a greeting, "Hey, Alicia, what's up?" Alicia snapped back, "Get out of here, you wretched skank!" Why? Because, she says, this girl had earlier glanced "flirtatiously" at Zach.

One day, after discussing these events, Alicia suddenly glared at me and asked, "Why doesn't anybody ever help me figure out what to do with my friends? Why don't you or my parents tell me how to handle stuff!" Alicia's complaint was right on target. Parents and even therapists, afraid of being oppressive, are often loath to offer clear, uncensored advice.

The following week, I told Alicia's parents that in order for Alicia's rage to cool down, she had to feel greater competence with her peers, and for this she needed their guidance. As usual, a straightforward directive to parents about *their* particular child triggered underlying family dynamics. Both Alicia's parents, Phyllis and Dean, grew up with terrible memories of overly critical and demanding parents who never gave them a moment's privacy or peace; their own laissez-faire approach toward Alicia was generated in the perfectly honorable desire not to squelch her personality. However, with my encouragement, one night, after Alicia yelled that she didn't want to hear anything about *her* life from *them* and ran into her room, Phyllis followed and waited outside the locked door. Phyllis was shocked when her daughter opened the door a crack and listened to what she had to say. Alicia was just as surprised that her mother actually pursued her to help.

So astonishing was the ensuing engagement between mother and daughter that Alicia began to share the incredible complexity of her social world with Phyllis, not to mention participating with her mother in some forays to local outlet stores. It wasn't long before she brought Zach to her house for Mom and Dad to meet (in order to get their opinion of him, she confided to me). Because Alicia felt guided at home, she was more adept with the other girls in class. She became less quick to lash out; she understood better how she hurt others' feelings and tried to actively repair ruptures when they did occur.

Just as strengthening one core skill in Jay and Eddie had a ripple effect leading to the improvement in other parts of their lives, so it was with Alicia. Feeling more confident with her peers, Alicia's grades soared, and she finished the year with a flurry of constructive activities—school projects, experimental writing, and community service camp. Alicia will never be a shrinking violet, and she can still make the air crackle with sharp witticisms. But, at 13, she is bursting out from behind her sardonic wall.

This has been increasingly the pattern with most of the children I see. What is most striking, however, are not the dramatic changes in their emotions and behavior but the fact that what worked with Alicia, Jay, and Eddie was not remotely interchangeable. The more these kids felt personally known and parented in ways that fit them, the less angry and dangerous their public statements became.

*   *   *

In a classroom discussion I led recently, 11-year-old Amanda made this stunning commentary: "If the adults [parents] don't know what's going on, it all turns into chaos." She could have been talking about professionals—therapists, counselors, teachers, doctors, clergy, and community leaders—as well. Although Amanda didn't realize it, she was describing the new paradigm. It is our job to know the facts of healthy child development. It is our responsibility to stand for something. It is our task to help parents learn who a child is and what he or she needs in order to develop a strong core self. For, as tragic events repeatedly demonstrate, we are in a life-and-death struggle over who will connect to the core selves of our children—mothers and fathers or the enveloping world of the second family.

"The adults need to know," says Amanda, the classroom becoming entirely still. And, for what seems like an endless and frighteningly intimate moment, all the children's eyes are fixed on the teacher and me.

Index